国际工程科技发展战略高端论坛

International Top-level Forum on Engineering
Science and Technology Development Strategy

中国工程院
CHINESE ACADEMY OF ENGINEERING

健康中国，策略为先

JIANKANG ZHONGGUO，CELUE WEIXIAN

STRATEGY AS A PRIORITY FOR THE HEALTHY CHINA INITIATIVE

高等教育出版社·北京

中国工程院

内容提要

本书是中国工程院国际工程科技发展战略高端论坛系列丛书之一。2017 年 11 月 18—19 日，由中国工程院主办，中国工程院工程管理学部、医药卫生学部和中华预防医学会共同承办的国际工程科技发展战略高端论坛——"健康中国"在北京召开。论坛以"公共卫生助力健康中国"为主题，围绕"把健康融入所有政策"，邀请了 6 位国内院士、3 位国际专家作了大会报告。国内专家从培育健康人群、优化健康服务、完善健康政策等角度，深刻阐释健康中国建设的理念、路径，分享中国智慧、中国案例；国外专家介绍了全球健康促进工作进展和成功经验，清晰解读了 2030 可持续发展目标中卫生与健康领域工作指标。本书收入了 8 位专家的报告全文。

本书适合从事卫生与健康领域工作的政府工作人员、科研院所研究人员及高校师生等阅读。

图书在版编目（CIP）数据

健康中国，策略为先：汉、英 ／ 中国工程院编著
. -- 北京：高等教育出版社,2019.5
（中国工程院"国际工程科技发展战略高端论坛"系列）
ISBN 978-7-04-051728-6

Ⅰ.①健… Ⅱ.①中… Ⅲ.①医疗保健事业-研究报
告-中国-汉、英 Ⅳ.①R199.2

中国版本图书馆 CIP 数据核字(2019)第 067193 号

总 策 划　樊代明

策划编辑　黄慧靖	责任编辑　张 冉	封面设计　顾 斌	版式设计　张 杰
插图绘制　于 博	责任校对　张 薇	责任印制　韩 刚	

出版发行　高等教育出版社	网　　址	http://www.hep.edu.cn
社　　址　北京市西城区德外大街 4 号		http://www.hep.com.cn
邮政编码　100120	网上订购	http://www.hepmall.com.cn
印　　刷　北京汇林印务有限公司		http://www.hepmall.com
开　　本　850 mm×1168 mm　1/16		http://www.hepmall.cn
印　　张　11		
字　　数　208 千字	版　　次	2019 年 5 月第 1 版
购书热线　010-58581118	印　　次	2019 年 5 月第 1 次印刷
咨询电话　400-810-0598	定　　价	80.00 元

目　录

CONTENTS

第一部分

综述

综　　述

王陇德　杨维中　刘　霞　田传胜　辛美哲
夏建国　杨　鹏　崔增伟

中华预防医学会

一、论坛整体情况

2017年11月18—19日,国际工程科技发展战略高端论坛——"健康中国"在北京盛大举行,大会的主题为"公共卫生助力健康中国"。来自中国工程院、中国科学技术协会(以下简称中国科协)、国家卫生和计划生育委员会(现为国家卫生健康委员会,以下简称国家卫生计生委)、各级医疗卫生机构、科研院所、高等院校、相关学(协)会的专家学者、专业技术人员及健康相关企业等共计2000余名代表参加了会议。

开幕式由中华预防医学会副会长兼秘书长杨维中主持。本次论坛主席、第十二届全国人大教科文卫委员会副主任委员、中华预防医学会会长、中国工程院院士王陇德,中国科协党组成员、学会学术部部长兼企业工作办公室主任宋军代表全国政协副主席、中国科协名誉主席韩启德,国家卫生计生委副主任、国家中医药管理局局长王国强,中国工程院副院长刘旭,世界公共卫生联盟主席Michael Moore,世界卫生组织驻华代表处官员Fabio Scano先后在开幕式上致辞,呼吁各界携手,坚持"预防为主"的工作方针,紧密对接并服务于健康中国战略,为推动我国"健康中国"的建设贡献力量。李兰娟院士、张伯礼院士以及相关单位的领导们出席了开幕式的中华预防医学会科学技术奖颁奖等环节。

本次论坛邀请到王陇德、刘旭、韦钰、陈君石、高润霖、钟南山6位中国工程院院士,以及Evelyne de Leeuw、Timo Stahl、Michael Moore 3位国际著名专家作大会报告。陈君石院士和陈育德教授、王宇研究员和Evelyne de Leeuw教授分别主持了上午和下午的会议。院士们围绕"把健康融入所有政策",从培育健康人群、优化健康服务、完善健康政策等角度,深刻阐释了健康中国建设的理念、路径,分享中国智慧、中国案例。几位国外专家介绍了全球健康促进工作的进展和成功经验,清晰解读了 2030 可持续发展目标中卫生与健康领域的工作指标。最后,大会主席王陇德院士做了会议闭幕总结。

与此会议同期召开的还有中华预防医学会第五届学术年会暨 2017 年中国慢性病大会。会议邀请 200 余位专家在 27 个分会场上作了专题报告,共组织论文交流 500 余篇,评选优秀论文近 50 篇。交流内容覆盖慢性病防治、卫生应急、健康评估与健康管理、健康促进与健康教育、疫苗与免疫、流行病学、生命早期发育与疾病控制、儿童成人病防治等健康领域热点难点问题。会议期间还颁发了 2017 年中华预防医学会科学技术奖、中华预防医学会系列杂志 2015—2016 年度优秀期刊奖和优秀期刊工作者奖;表彰了中国慢性病防控最佳实践案例、"健康中国·科普中国——全国慢性病防治优秀科普作品推介工程"首届活动优秀科普图书、首届全国妈妈班优秀科普视频;发布了《中国公共卫生与预防医学学科史》《2049 年的中国:科技与社会愿景——预防医学与生命质量》《2016 年中国人口健康状况报告》3 个征求意见稿;平行召开了中国妇女盆底功能障碍防治项目总结暨表彰会。

本次论坛是在党的十九大胜利闭幕后不久,落实十九大报告中明确提出的"要实施健康中国战略"而召开的一次盛会。会议得到健康领域各级机构和专业人员的高度重视。全国政协副主席韩启德专门为大会发表书面讲话。100 多家中外机构发来贺信贺电,10 位院士给予题词或寄语。新华社、健康报、科技日报、人民网、光明网、中国网、央广网、央视网等 20 多家媒体进行了现场报道;还通过中华预防医学会官网和官微、光明网等平台进行了大会直播,并邀请到 6 位院士、10 余位权威专家参与健康领域热点科普在线访谈直播,直播浏览量达 110 多万人次。

二、专家发言及研讨内容

大会主席、中华预防医学会会长王陇德院士作了题为"健康中国,策略当先"的报告。他指出,当前中国,健康领域改革发展取得了显著成就,人民健康水平和身体素质持续提高,但健康服务供给总体不足与需求不断增长之间的矛盾依然突出,健康领域发展与经济社会发展的协调性有待增强,需要从国家战略层面统筹解决关系健康的重大问题和长远问题。国家为此明确要"实施健康中国战略",完善国民健康政策,为人民群众提供全方位全周期健康服务;《"健康中国 2030"规划纲要》也提出了两阶段的发展战略目标和一系列的具体指标、要求。王院士还分享了推进"把健康融入所有政策"立法以及在卫生技术策略、适宜技术普及等方面的一些策略探索实践与体会。

中国工程院副院长刘旭院士在题为"农业、食物发展与国民营养健康"的报告中,分析了当前我国食物供给与消费的变化趋势及其与健康的关系,建议可主要从农业供给侧、需求侧和宏观调控三个方面着手,来促进农业发展和国民营养健康改善:从农业供给层面,仍要继续增加食物总量、改善质量;从需求侧层面,要推进膳食指南的落实,新增若干食物的消费补贴和食物援助,对食物消费进行监测和引导;从宏观调控层面,各级政府要强化对食物营养工作的指导和保障。

原国家教育部副部长韦钰院士在题为"遵循脑发展的规律,培养健康和优秀的下一代"的报告中强调,从孕期到幼儿3岁之间,是人发展过程中的重要时期。在这个阶段,既存在着促进人生发展的良好机遇,又是对遭受不同困境儿童产生严重不良影响的敏感期。不仅是营养不良和各种侵害会引起严重的后果,即使是忽视和冷漠的教养环境,也会对儿童造成很大的伤害,从而改变他们脑发育和发展过程,影响一生的健康状况,增加患病概率,降低认知能力。因此建议将国家扶贫关注的时间点前移到生命早期1000天,整合医疗、教育和各方面的扶贫力量,支持和改善困境儿童家庭教养的质量,实施帮助困境儿童的整合行动。这也是提高精准扶贫、实现教育公平、阻断贫困代际传递的有效措施。

国家食品安全风险评估中心的陈君石院士作了题为"营养助力健康中国"的报告,指出营养与国人的健康和疾病密切相关,实施《"健康中国2030"规划纲要》,全面建成小康社会,离不开营养学。他从解读国际、国内最新健康政策和《"健康中国2030"规划纲要》等文件入手,分析了《国民营养计划(2017—2030年)》出台的背景,指出营养与健康正面临最好的政策时代,相信相关计划的落实和实施一定会对全面建成小康社会和实现健康中国梦做出重要贡献。

国家心血管病中心高润霖院士作了题为"中国心血管病的现状和防治策略"的报告,指出心血管病是我国城乡居民的第一位死亡原因,且死亡率仍呈上升趋势。心血管病死亡率上升主要由于人口老龄化和危险因素流行,高血压、高胆固醇血症、糖尿病、吸烟、超重肥胖等是最重要的危险因素。防治心血管病的关键是防控危险因素,政府主导,预防为主,规范防治管理落地,建立分级诊疗制度,推动"医疗保障"向"健康保障"转型,充分发挥"互联网+"的作用。"把健康融入所有政策",加强各行业、各部门沟通协作,"三高共管",将对我国心血管病防治早日达到死亡率下降拐点起到巨大作用。

广州医科大学教授、国家呼吸系统疾病临床医学研究中心主任钟南山院士作了题为"健康中国——呼吸系统疾病早诊早治战略"的报告,从占据我国总死亡人数11%的慢性呼吸系统疾病入手,指出其三大主要影响因素是严重的空气污染、吸烟和频发重大急性呼吸系统传染病，并以肺癌和慢阻肺诊断控制为实例，阐述了应贯彻落实我国健康与卫生工作的方针，实现疾病临床防治的早期预防、早期干预。

《国际健康促进》杂志主编 Evelyne de Leeuw 教授作了题为"卫生政策综合协调的原因和举措"的报告。她重点强调了健康是受多种因素影响的，同样，将健康融入所有政策也是受不同的社会因素影响的。

芬兰国家公共卫生研究院 Timo Stahl 教授介绍了"芬兰'把健康融入所有政策'的成功实践"。在报告中，Stahl 教授重点介绍了 2007 年由芬兰在欧盟提出的"把健康融入所有政策"的历史、"把健康融入所有政策"的具体做法以及经验教训。他们得到的经验教训是，首先要有长期的投入和规划，"把健康融入所有政策"不会一蹴而就，需要公共卫生和沟通方面的专业知识；需要所有人的参与，不仅需要临床医生的参与，还需要其他人的参与；需要有数据，要整合关于健康和健康决定因素的数据，来分析健康的结果、健康决定因素和政策之间的联系；需要提高公共机构、决策者、媒体、公务人员的健康素养，还需要跨部门的结构流程和工具，来使得"把健康融入所有政策"更加系统化。这些工具可以帮助我们认识问题、解决问题，并做出决策以及部署部门间的行动。芬兰的实践证明，"立法支持"是非常有用的。

世界公共卫生联盟主席 Michael Moore 博士在题为"2030 更健康：《全球公共卫生宪章》与可持续发展目标"的报告中，重点介绍了世界公共卫生联盟与世界卫生组织以及包括许多国际非政府组织在内的利益攸关方合作制定的《全球公共卫生宪章》（以下简称《宪章》）。《宪章》作为协助落实联合国可持续发展目标的途径，旨在摆脱以疾病为中心的政策，并通过"预防、保护和健康促进"为改善健康提供指导，其四大推动力是"能力建设、良好的治理、信息和宣传"。报告结合联合国可持续发展目标中的一些例子（譬如保护人类健康不受气候风险影响，通过低碳发展促进健康；负责任的消费和生产；优先考虑穷人的健康需求，减少不平等；良好健康与福祉；清洁用水和卫生设施以及健康伙伴关系等）说明了如何利用《宪章》的关键因素，采取一系列更加切实的措施，结合"把健康融入所有政策"，为可持续发展目标创造更好的健康成果。

这些专家来自不同的行业和领域，具有极高的学术造诣，具有在多个重要部门和机构的高层管理经验，他们聚焦"健康中国"主题，从健康立法、强化国民营养、关注儿童早期发育、实施心血管病和呼吸系统疾病早诊早治战略等方面进行报告，并分享了全球健康促进工作的最新进展和成功经验，强调政府主导、部门合作、全社会参与，深刻阐释了推动健康中国建设的理念、路径，提出了针对性强、具体可操作的政策建议,极大地提升了论坛的学术影响力,也形成了包括行政部门领导在内的所有与会者的强烈共识,必将促进"把健康融入所有政策"的强大合力的形成和增强。

第二部分
致辞

致　辞

刘　旭

中国工程院

尊敬的王陇德会长、王国强副主任、宋军部长,各位院士,各位中外来宾,女士们、先生们:

大家上午好!

今天,由中国工程院主办的"健康中国"国际工程科技发展战略高端论坛在京隆重召开,我谨代表中国工程院,代表周济院长,向出席论坛的中外嘉宾表示热烈的欢迎! 向参与组织论坛的中华预防医学会等有关单位和人员表示衷心的感谢!

健康是人类永恒的话题,人民健康是民族昌盛和国家富强的重要标志。习近平总书记高度重视人民健康,他明确指出,没有全民健康,就没有全面小康。"健康中国"是以习近平同志为核心的党中央提出的新时代奋斗目标。2015 年党的十八届五中全会首次将"健康中国"上升为国家战略;2016 年新世纪第一次全国卫生与健康大会召开,出台了《"健康中国 2030"规划纲要》;2017 年党的十九大报告中再次明确"实施健康中国战略",提出了"要完善国民健康政策,为人民群众提供全方位全周期健康服务"的新时代要求。这些充分展示了国家将人民健康提升到了前所未有的高度。

中国工程院是中国工程科技界最高荣誉性、咨询性学术机构,是中国工程科技思想库。为切实发挥思想库作用,加强学术引领,紧密对接并服务于健康中国战略,我们主办本次国际工程科技发展战略高端论坛,聚焦"健康中国",邀请国内外顶尖专家就健康主题进行交流研讨,交流最新进展,分享先进理念,凝聚广泛共识,为推动健康中国建设贡献力量。

本次论坛得到了众多院士、专家的高度关注和大力支持,6 位来自不同领域的国内院士将围绕"把健康融入所有政策",从培育健康人群、优化健康服务、完善健康政策等角度,深刻阐释健康中国建设的理念、路径,分享中国智慧、中国案例；几位国外知名专家将为我们带来全球健康促进工作进展和成功经验，清晰解读 2030 可持续发展目标中卫生与健康领域工作指标。这些精彩的报告对于我们更加牢固地树立"大健康、大卫生"观念，必将起到积极的促进作用。

同志们，朋友们，这场学术盛宴即将开启，希望大家能畅所欲言、深入研讨，为推动我国"健康中国"的建设积极建言献策，为实现全民健康做出新的更大的贡献！

最后，衷心祝愿本次论坛取得圆满成功！祝愿大家工作顺利，身体健康！

谢谢大家！

第三部分
主题报告

健康中国,策略当先

王陇德

中华预防医学会

今天我想从以下三个方面和大家做讨论:一是健康中国战略制定的国内外背景,以便我们更好地理解健康中国战略的主要内涵;二是健康中国战略的主要内容和发展目标;三是向大家汇报下我们关于一些重点目标实现的策略探索和体会。

一、健康中国战略制定的背景

在国内,多年来健康领域的改革取得了显著成效,人民健康水平和身体素质持续提高。但工业化、人口老龄化、生态环境和生活方式的变化也给我们的健康带来了一系列的挑战。

营养不良和母婴疾病在明显减少,但超重肥胖这样的慢性病主要危险因素大幅度地增加,所以我国的慢性病发病人数快速上升。慢性病造成的死亡率占总死亡率的比例已经上升到了85%以上,其中心脑血管病造成的死亡率占慢性病死亡率的50%以上。

国际上特别重视慢性病对人类的危害。2011年,第66届联合国大会召开了慢性病防控高级别会议,提出政府各级要制定多部门的卫生工作方针。2015年,联合国193个成员国通过了联合国的2030可持续发展议程。议程里明确提出了17项关于可持续发展的目标,几乎每项目标都和健康有着密切的关系,特别是目标2、目标3、目标6明确提出健康相关要求。

世界卫生组织也从1986年起组织全球健康促进大会,到2013年已经召开了8届,每一届都提出了健康促进需要推进的一些重要工作:1986年明确了健康促进的五大新领域,1988年提出了制定健康的公共政策,1991年提出了创造健康的支持性环境等重要内涵。

2016年,第九届全球健康促进大会在我国上海举办,这次大会的主题是"可持续发展中的健康促进"，就是探讨怎样更好地吻合联合国的可持续发展目标。

我国制定健康中国战略也有一个比较好的基础。那就是2008年，当时的陈竺部长提出了健康中国2020战略研究，目的是提高城乡居民健康状况，改善国民健康总质量。该研究提出了两步走的工作方针，提出了12项目标（主要包括提高预期寿命、缩小地区差异、发展健康产业、履行政府职责等），同时也提出了10项实现这些目标的具体政策建议，以保障国民健康水平的进一步提高。

以上我简单介绍了健康中国战略制定的背景。

二、健康中国战略的主要内容和发展目标

首先是党的十八届五中全会明确了这一宏伟战略。同时，在2016年召开的第一次全国卫生与健康大会上，习近平总书记代表中央明确了新时期的卫生与健康工作方针。该方针和以往的卫生工作方针最大的区别在于明确了"把健康融入所有政策"。会后，中共中央政治局又审议通过了《"健康中国2030"规划纲要》（以下简称《纲要》）。这是今后15年推进健康中国建设的行动纲领。党的十九大报告也再次明确了要实施健康中国战略，为人民群众提供全方位、全周期的健康服务。

那么《纲要》有哪些要点？首先，提出了四项主要原则：① 健康优先；② 改革创新，形成具有中国特色、促进全民健康的制度体系；③ 科学发展，就是要坚持预防为主、防治结合，提升健康服务水平；④ 公平公正，逐步缩小城乡、地区、人群间基本健康服务和健康水平的差异。同时，也提出了战略主题——"共建共享，全民健康"。共建共享是建设健康中国的基本路径，从供给侧和需求侧两端发力；全民健康是建设健康中国的根本目的。

战略发展目标分为两个阶段：到2020年，主要健康指标要居于中高收入国家前列；到2030年，主要健康指标要进入高收入国家行列。

《纲要》还提出了一些具体的指标，涉及五个方面13项具体要实现的指标，包括人均期望寿命、居民健康素养水平、健康服务业总规模等。这里，我想具体谈谈有关健康期望寿命的问题。

原来是以期望寿命代表一个国家的国民健康水平。而现在人类的重大问题是活得长了，但是不是活得健康、活得幸福？21世纪初，世界卫生组织新提出了"健康期望寿命"这样一个指标。主要发达国家的期望寿命和健康期望寿命间大约相差10岁，但我国目前为止还没有条件去测算全国居民的健康期望寿命。有些地方，在局部地区做了些研究，例如北京，2012年做了一个北京市居民的健康期望寿命评估，评估结果是北京市的居民健康期望寿命与期望寿命居然相差20

岁。而且,一个北京市的居民即使在 18 岁时很健康,也不一定能活到 60 岁。这是我国目前面临的一个重大问题,就是慢性病年轻化趋势。我们虽然尚不具备测算全国居民健康期望寿命的条件,但我们不能永远不具备。我们是不是至少在 2020 年之前能够创造条件测算我国居民的健康期望寿命? 所以我们在《纲要》里提出了一个新目标,就是到 2030 年国民健康期望寿命有显著增长。

三、重点目标实现的策略探索和体会

关于推进重点目标,给大家介绍一些相关的体会。重要的目标,一定要有重点的策略来推进其实现。那么首先我们得研究重点问题。在实现健康中国建设目标方面存在哪些重点问题? 首先是全社会的协同缺乏。政府各部门协同、全社会参与的局面还没有形成。其次,还有一个基础的问题——国民健康素养低下,特别是慢性病危险因素广泛流行,吸烟、酗酒这样的不健康行为非常普遍。再次,还有工作上的问题,我们的服务体系不适应居民健康的需求。在慢性病流行为主的年代,要控制慢性病,医疗机构的参与是非常重要的。但我国的医疗机构绝大部分仅仅还是做疾病诊疗,等发病后才参与,而很少参与危险因素的筛查和控制。所以从这个意义上来说,我们慢性病防控体系的建设仅仅处于一个起步阶段。这造成了我国心脑血管病、高血压、血脂异常、高血糖的控制率非常低。

再谈谈国民第一位死因——脑卒中(又称“中风”)的流行情况。最近几年的脑卒中研究数据分析结果证明了我们现在的卒中患者几乎 50% 是中年人,而中年人的发病、死亡以及造成的残疾给家庭和社会造成的影响非常严重。根据预测,如果我们这种局面不改变,那么会从现在的 1100 万到 1200 万的脑卒中患者发展到 2030 年的 3100 万。此外还分析了卒中高危人群的年龄比例,中年人居然占到了 60%。我们觉得这个问题是影响国民健康最重要的因素之一,因此给中央写了一份院士建议,习近平总书记、刘延东副总理做出了批示,要求开展中年人脑卒中危险因素的筛查和控制。

对于重点问题,我们要采取什么策略? 我们觉得应该从以下几方面采取工作。

(一) 明确职责,立法保障

首先应该明确职责。中央已经明确了要求,那么怎么实现? 首先要明确政府相关部委的职责,国家层面上必须建立慢性病防控的工作体系,把医疗机构逐步纳入工作体系中;国家还应该明确重点和目标、设立示范项目来引导各地区的工作。例如财政部,是不是应该研究政府购买服务的政策? 要提高群众健康水平,实现分级诊疗是非常重要的措施。但分级诊疗的实现必须首先提高基层医务工作者的水平，把问题给老百姓解决在基层。但我们目前的基层服务能力非常欠缺，那就必须由上级医疗专家下去培训。上级医疗机构专家下基层，谁来保障费用？我们现在是安排任务，让医院自己解决，实际上是不可持续的。所以我们的政府怎样为这项工作来买单？作为临床医务工作者，以前你会诊疗疾病就是合格的医务工作者，现在到了慢性病流行的年代，仅仅会这些已经不是合格的医务人员了。每个临床工作者必须了解重大慢性病的防控知识和技能，必须在自己的工作岗位上开展慢性病防控。我们要提高国民的健康素养，宣传也是个很重要的工作领域。怎样发动宣传部门，让他们能够把健康科普知识的宣传作为他们的主要任务？当然这还需要政府给予相关的资金支持。

对于医保部门来说，目前的政策是报销疾病发生后的治疗费用和重病抢救费用，很少支付慢性病危险因素控制费用。而发达国家已经发展到对于具有慢性危险因素，像超重、肥胖，甚至健身锻炼都纳入医保。所以我们是否应重新研究相关政策？

我们要提高健康素养，必须得从小教起，从小培养孩子，使他们在孩童阶段就形成健康的生活方式和习惯，同时也教给孩子的家长。在这一方面，教育部门责无旁贷。另外，民政部门也不能只管发结婚证，他们可以进一步为申请结婚登记的青年男女提供关于优生和科学育儿的知识培训。哪对新婚夫妇不希望生出个健康的孩子，不希望自己的孩子健康成长？

我记得，二三十年前，很多单位、企业都有医务室，现在基本全没了。职能社区的所有成员有健康问题都到三级医疗机构看病，使三级医疗机构不堪重负。我们职工有没有体检，是否发现了威胁他们健康的主要危险因素？单位食堂健康食品制作得怎么样，是不是高盐、高糖、高油？单位、企业是否应该设专人负责这些问题？我们的一些社会团体，比如妇联，能不能做些关于健康膳食的培训？女性在家庭中的地位非常重要，她做什么饭，家里就吃什么，她做的食物健康了，家庭健康就基本有了保证。目前我们正在努力在卫生法的制定过程中争取把这些健康保障写进去，以保证"把健康融入所有政策"的原则的实现。

（二）提高素养，造就基础

世界卫生组织总结全球研究结果表明，人们的生活方式和行为对寿命和健康的影响占了60%。而现在我们的健康素养非常低，10个人里只有1个人掌握基本的健康素养。因此，如果不改变这样的状态，慢性病的流行是无法控制的。

（三）防控危因，狠抓关键

美国总结了近50年来脑卒中死亡率、发病率不断下降的经验，控制血压、血脂、血糖以及戒烟等是主要的原因，其中控制血压是最主要的原因，如果血压控制得好，近一半的中风可以不发病。但我国国民的血压知晓率、控制率、治疗率还很低，很多农村居民没有量过血压。很多高血压患者也没有吃药，他们不明白高血压巨大的风险在哪里。这几年我们采取了一些措施，动员了318家三甲医院参与到卒中防控工程中来，这些医院又联系了1000多家医院作为协作单位，联系了2700多家社区乡镇卫生机构做筛查控制。同时在这项工作中，我们也探索了一个防控技术策略——32字方针：关口前移、重心下沉、提高素养、宣教先行、学科合作、规范防治、高危筛查、目标干预。

在这项工作中，我们推广适宜技术，并编写教材。在全国选了20多家三甲医院，近几年培训了11万医务人员，同时对一些适宜的技术做推广。例如颈动脉严重狭窄，其是引发卒中的重要原因之一。我们2010年做了多少CEA（颈动脉内膜剥脱术）手术？247例。这些年来我们重点推广CEA手术这样的防控技术，最近几年每年已经实施3000多例。发达国家卒中患者的溶栓率达到20%~30%，而我国不到2%。不要说县级医疗机构，绝大部分的三级医疗机构都没有很好地开展溶栓，所以患者的残疾率非常高。按道理讲，一个医院只要有了CT就能够开展这项工作。我们的县级及以上医院均有CT，但这项技术以往却没有被推广。这些年我们在大力推广这些技术。以前三级医院的患者溶栓得2个小时，而国际上的要求是1个小时。近些年我们也在进行服务程序的改革，限定溶栓每一个阶段的时间。超出规定时间，工作就不合格。现在很多卒中防治基地医院已经把溶栓的时间缩短到了1个小时之内。

下一步我们的重点工作是一定要建立卒中的1小时黄金急救圈；要建立地区防控网络。仅靠国家一级的防控网络和项目，每年只能筛查100万40岁以上的人口。仅靠国家网络，广泛的群众受益得等到什么时候？所以国家的卒中综合防治方案里明确提出目标，就是要建立卒中的地区医疗防控网络，到2020年前一定要建成，1小时黄金救治圈也要建成。

（四）组建体系，创新模式

要组建的体系，就是健康教育体系。这项工作仅仅靠卫生部门是不行的，必须得靠广电、宣传、教育等多部门的协同。习总书记也提出了要建立健全健康教育体系，要用人民群众听得到、听得懂、听得进的方式传播健康知识。

（五）监察督察，力求实效

以前中央提出的一些原则没有很好地实现，就是因为没有督促检查，所以《"健康中国 2030"规划纲要》对监测、评估、督察提出了明确要求。

相信我们在政府主导、多部门合作、全社会参与的工作机制下，落实"把健康融入所有政策"，就一定能更有效地凝聚全社会之力，推动健康中国建设的目标早日实现。

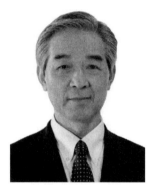

王陇德　中国工程院院士，中华预防医学会会长，第十二届全国人大常委会委员、教科文卫委员会副主任委员。原国家卫生部党组副书记、副部长。兼任国家卫生计生委疾病预防控制专家委员会主任委员、健康促进与教育专家指导委员会主任委员、脑卒中筛查与防治工程委员会副主任、科技创新战略顾问等职。

他长期在公共卫生领域从事行政管理、流行病学和公众健康促进专业研究工作。提出并领导组建了全国医疗机构传染病和突发公共卫生事件网络直报系统；研究提出了以控制传染源为主的血吸虫病控制新策略；提出并组织实施了全国"脑卒中筛查与防治工程"。在《新英格兰医学杂志》等国内外学术期刊发表论文百余篇，主编多部专著。获国家科技进步奖二等奖、联合国艾滋病规划署应对艾滋病杰出领导和持续贡献奖、世界卫生组织结核病控制高川奖和世界卫生组织世界无烟日奖等。

农业、食物发展与国民营养健康

刘　旭

中国工程院

今天主要从以下四个方面,与大家共同探讨"农业、食物发展与国民营养健康"这个话题。一是当前我国农业生产与食物供给现状;二是居民食物消费特点与趋势;三是居民营养与健康状况;四是农业发展与国民营养健康改善的建议。

一、当前我国农业生产与食物供给现状

(一)当前我国农业生产现状

一是各类食用农产品生产水平高并呈稳定态势。2016年,我国粮食产量6.16亿t,其中稻谷2.07亿t、小麦1.29亿t、玉米2.20亿t,与2015年相比下降0.8%,粮食总量"十二连增"后首次小幅回落。2016年,动物产品总产量2.21亿t,其中肉、蛋、奶、水产品总产量分别为8540万t、3095万t、3602万t、6900万t,与2015年基本持平。2016年,蔬菜、水果总产量在10亿t以上,保持2015年生产水平。

二是农业生产条件逐步改善。2015年,全国农业机械总动力11亿kW,农作物耕种收综合机械化率为63%。主要作物薄弱环节机械化快速推进,2015年水稻种植、玉米收获机械化率分别超过40%、63%,分别比"十一五"末提高19个百分点、37个百分点。2015年,按照城镇由大到小、空间由近及远、耕地质量由高到低的顺序,全面开展永久基本农田划定工作,106个重点城市周边永久基本农田划定工作取得积极进展。农机社会化服务向纵深发展,由耕—种—收环节向产前—产中—产后全环节加快拓展,农机专业合作社超过5.65万个,全程机械化服务能力明显增强。

三是食物加工产能快速增长。改革开放以来,我国农产品加工业产值年均增长速度超过13%,明显高于同期GDP增长速度。截至2014年,农产品加工企业

达 45.5 万家,其中规模以上企业 7.6 万家,实现主营业务收入 18.48 万亿元,利润总额达到 1.22 万亿元,农产品加工业与农业产值比达到 2.1∶1。以粮油、肉类、奶类、果蔬以及特色资源食品为重点的产业集群式发展格局逐步形成,新兴方便食品、休闲食品、绿色食品等市场份额继续扩大,调理食品、保健食品等功能性食品逐步受到消费者认可。

（二）当前国内农业及食物有效供给的总体状况

一是从质量安全保障即"吃得放心"上看,随着我国农业综合生产能力的提升和农业对外开放的扩大,我国食物质量安全水平稳中有升。食用农产品抽检总体合格率连续多年稳定在 96% 以上,保持了总体平稳、持续向好的态势。2015 年,全年农产品质量总体合格率为 97.1%,蔬菜、水果、茶叶、畜禽产品和水产品例行监测合格率分别为 96.1%、95.6%、97.6%、99.4% 和 95.5%。2015 年,全国绿色食品产地环境监测面积为 2.6 亿亩（1 亩 ≈ 666.67 m^2）,与 2000 年相比,增加约 3.5 倍。

二是从供给数量保障即"吃饱""吃好"上看,当前我国食物生产及有效供给能够满足居民对食物营养的保障需求。在 2015 年国内食物总供给水平下,扣除损耗和不可食部分,我国各类食物每日人均可提供热量 2855 kcal、蛋白质 103 g、脂肪 77 g,与发达国家水平较为接近。中国每日人均热量、蛋白质、脂肪需求量分别为 1910 kcal、67 g、58 g。从三大营养素分析,中国食物生产及有效供给能够满足国内居民的健康营养需求。

三是从食物供求平衡状况看,我国食物自给水平总体较高,国内食物种类"供大于求"与"供不足需"并存,个别品种供大于求,这也是当前及今后一段时期我国农业供给侧结构急需调整的主要缘由。

二、居民食物消费特点与趋势

从食物结构分析,30 多年来我国居民食物消费的变化态势表现在以下三个方面。

一是年人均口粮消费量逐步下降,其中城镇居民的人均消费量呈较稳定的态势。1981 年以来,城乡居民人均口粮消费量（按原粮计）基本呈逐步下降态势,农村人均消费量由 260 kg 减少到 176 kg,城镇居民人均消费量由 201 kg 下降到 2009 年的 139 kg,之后保持相对稳定。

二是年人均动物产品消费量呈增长态势,但城乡消费差距依然较大。1981—2015 年,城乡居民人均动物产品消费量（按原粮计）均呈上升态势,农村人均消费量由 12.2 kg 增加到 57.5 kg,城镇居民人均消费量由 37.1 kg 提高至 106.1 kg。城乡居民动物产品消费差距绝对量在扩大,但相对差距在缩小,城乡消费比由 3∶1 减少为 1.8∶1。

三是人均蔬菜消费量整体趋减,但城镇居民的减幅相对较小。1981—2015 年,农村人均消费量由 126.0 kg 减少到 98.1 kg,下降了约 1/5;城镇居民由 152.3 kg 减少为 139.3 kg,下降幅度不到 10%。

对我国未来食物消费总体趋势做一个判断:目前,我国城乡居民恩格尔系数已分别降低到 36.2%、39.3%。按照联合国粮食及农业组织(FAO)发布的标准判断,我国经济社会发展已进入相对富裕阶段。从消费模式相似的区域变化规律来看,当居民恩格尔系数处于 20%～40% 的发展阶段,未来我国居民膳食结构升级的主要特征趋势判断为:口粮逐渐下降、动物产品消费有所增长,并将带动食物消费总需求的缓慢上升。

三、国民营养与健康状况

从国民营养状况来分析,一是 30 多年来国民热量摄入量逐步减少;二是国民蛋白质摄入量总体稳定;三是国民蛋白摄入量中的动物蛋白占比明显提高;四是国民脂肪摄入量总体趋增,这是肥胖等营养性疾病高发的主要诱因。

从国民健康状况来分析,一是儿童、青少年生长迟缓率降低。与 2002 年相比,2010—2012 年我国 6～17 岁儿童、青少年的生长迟缓率降低了 3.1 个百分点,降幅 49%。二是各类人群贫血率明显下降。与 2002 年相比,2010—2012 年城乡不同性别、不同年龄段人群贫血患病率大幅下降,比较而言,农村居民降幅较大。三是成年人中的超重和肥胖人数不断增加。2012 年,全国成年人超重率为 30%、肥胖率为 12%,与 1992 年相比,分别高出 18 个百分点、8 个百分点。四是成年人糖尿病患病率呈"井喷"式上升。2012 年,全国成年人糖尿病患病率增加至 9.7%,与 2002 年相比,增加了 1 倍还多。

"民以食为天",食物营养是人类维持生命、生长发育和健康的重要物质基础,事关国民素质提高和经济社会发展。吃饱、吃好、吃得营养是维持健康的首要前提。但影响健康的有遗传、心理、生态环境、市场竞争等多种因素。这也是国家相继提出《"健康中国 2030"规划纲要》《国民营养计划(2017—2030 年)》《中国食物与营养发展纲要(2014—2020 年)》的主要缘由。

《"健康中国 2030"规划纲要》着重提出:"以提高人民健康水平为核心,以体制机制改革创新为动力,以普及健康生活、优化健康服务、完善健康保障、建设健康环境、发展健康产业为重点,把健康融入所有政策,加快转变健康领域发展方式,全方位、全周期维护和保障人民健康,大幅提高健康水平,显著改善健康公平";同时着重提出要"制定实施国民营养计划","推行健康生活方式",把"引导合理膳食"作为"塑造自主自律的健康行为"的首要措施。

《国民营养计划(2017—2030年)》着重提出:坚持以人民健康为中心,以普及营养健康知识、优化营养健康服务、完善营养健康制度、建设营养健康环境、发展营养健康产业为重点,立足现状,着眼长远,关注国民生命全周期、健康全过程的营养健康,将营养融入所有健康政策,不断满足人民群众营养健康需求,提高全民健康水平,为建设健康中国奠定坚实基础。

《中国食物与营养发展纲要2014—2020年》着重提出:一方面,近年来我国农产品综合生产能力稳步提高,食物供需基本平衡,食品安全状况总体稳定向好,居民营养健康状况明显改善,食物与营养发展成效显著;而另一方面,我国食物生产还不能适应营养需求,居民营养不足与过剩并存问题突出,还有数千万贫困人口及低收入人口的基本营养保障急需解决,人群中营养与健康知识严重缺乏,这些问题必须引起高度重视。

习近平总书记在党的十九大报告中强调指出:坚决打赢脱贫攻坚战。确保到2020年我国现行标准下农村贫困人口实现脱贫,贫困县全部摘帽,解决区域性整体贫困,做到脱真贫、真脱贫。实施乡村振兴战略。确保国家粮食安全,把中国人的饭碗牢牢端在自己手中。实施健康中国战略。人民健康是民族昌盛和国家富强的重要标志。坚持预防为主,深入开展爱国卫生运动,倡导健康文明生活方式,预防控制重大疾病。实施食品安全战略。让人民吃得放心。

四、关于农业发展与国民营养健康改善的建议

从农业供给侧层面,仍要继续增加食物总量、改善质量。一是提高粮食产量。根据人口增长对食物的需求预测,到2035年中国基本实现现代化时,总人口将达到15亿左右,年人均粮食消费量将达到450~470 kg,粮食总消费量7亿t左右,也就是说,粮食产量应该增加近1亿t才能满足需求。二是调整生产结构,增加优质比重、实行粮改饲。提高优质粳稻、强弱筋小麦、青贮玉米等产品比重,确保国内生产从数量与品质结构上与需求相匹配。三是改善食物品质。加快优质动植物种质资源开发和应用推广,改进提升传统农产品作坊式"土法"加工工艺水平,提升食用农产品的品质及营养功能。四是发展营养强化产品。研究表明,通过摄入食物获取的营养素,往往不能满足人体的所有需求。通过摄入相关的膳食补充剂和营养强化食品来满足人体的健康需求,正在成为新常态。

从需求侧层面,要推进膳食指南的落实,新增若干食物的消费补贴和食物援

助,对食物消费进行监测和引导。一是推动 2016 版《中国居民膳食指南》的落实、落地。通过电视、网络等主流媒体,建立膳食营养知识宣传普及的主渠道。建议借鉴国外做法,征收高糖、高脂等食品的消费税,在全国推行"全民减盐行动"、食用油"减油"行动以及控糖、限酒活动,保护消费者免受不健康食品的影响,并将税收用于公共卫生设施条件的改善。采取补贴措施将新鲜水果和蔬菜价格降低 10%～30%,促进居民蔬果消费。设立生物强化重大专项,加大对优质高产、高适应性生物强化研发及其产业化的支持力度。二是针对贫困、低收入群体进行食物援助。食物消费既是一个经济问题,也是一个社会问题,即使是食物供给十分充足的国家,也存在少数低收入人群食物安全基本供给问题。按照每人每年 2300 元(2010 年不变价)的农村贫困标准计算,2016 年我国还有农村贫困人口 4335 万人,普遍存在膳食摄入量不足、微量营养素缺乏等问题。建议国家应尽快组织发放"食物券",为贫困、低收入人群及中小学生提供基本营养需要,在老少边穷地区中小学校实施免费午餐行动;在贫困地区推行营养型农业发展,重点开发特色优质食物资源、新食品原料生产。三是建立居民食物消费监测与引导平台。建立不同区域以县级为单位的集食物生产、居民食物消费、营养教育于一体的观测站点。以计算机网络系统和移动通信等技术平台为依托,创建居民膳食质量在线评价工具,为实现膳食质量自我评价提供支撑。针对重点人群,设计个性化营养食谱和营养补充方案。研究居民食物消费行为影响因素,提出有针对性的消费引导与营养干预政策。

从宏观调控层面,各级政府要强化对食物营养工作的指导和保障。一是加快对食物营养的立法工作,把对重点地区重点人群实施营养干预,加强对学校、幼儿园、养老机构等营养健康工作的指导,保障低收入人群的基本营养需要作为各级政府和部门营养促进及干预的职责,推进食物与营养的法制化管理。二是贯彻落实《国民营养计划(2017—2030 年)》,构建农业、卫生与教育、科技、扶贫等部门的协调机制,推动食物与营养事业发展。三是将居民营养安全列入国家"十三五"发展目标。立足各地资源条件和消费习惯,提出不同地区不同人群膳食模式,将当地居民食物营养与健康状况纳入政府考核指标。

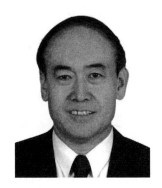

刘旭　中国工程院院士，植物种质资源学家。曾任中国工程院党组成员、副院长、机关党委书记，中国农业科学院党组成员、副院长。参与组织、领导了"中国农作物种质资源收集保存评价与利用""中国农作物种质资源本底多样性和技术指标体系及应用"等多项研究。组织与主持出版了《中国作物及其野生近缘植物》系列专著8卷、《中国农作物种质资源技术规范》系列110册。获国家、省部级科技进步奖多项。参与组织了国家农作物基因资源与基因改良重大工程筹建、国家基础性工作及国家自然科技资源共享平台的发展战略研究并组织实施。

遵循脑发展的规律，培养健康和优秀的下一代

韦　钰

中国工程院

习近平总书记十分关心贫困地区儿童的发展和教育工作，指出"扶贫必扶智"，强调要"阻止贫困现象代际传递"。2016 年，教育部与国家发展和改革委员会等六部门联合颁发了我国首个教育脱贫攻坚五年规划，采取了有效措施，在落实教育扶贫和教育公平上取得了很大的进展。党的十九大报告中，首次提出"幼有所育"这个新概念。在十九大精神的鼓舞下，我们应该借助科技的力量，将精确扶贫的工作做得更好。

现在大家对国民健康状况和相关疾病的预防十分重视。但是，健康并不只是躯体器官（如心、肺、肝等）的健康，还应该考虑脑的健康、精神的健康，甚至可以说，脑的健康比躯体健康更为重要，因为人之所以为人，你之所以为你，是因为你有一个独特的、强大的大脑。

在 1946 年世界卫生组织成立时的宪章里，给出了关于健康的定义：

"Health is a state of complete physical, mental and social well-being and not merely the absence of disease or infirmity."

对这个健康的定义有不同的中文译本，下面是两个通用的译法，都强调了健康不只是指躯体的健康，还应该包括心理和社会行为的完好状态，只是我们经常忽视了这个重要的内容，甚至遗忘了。

译法一：健康不仅是疾病与体虚的匿迹，而是身心健康和社会幸福的总体状况。

译法二：健康不仅是没有疾病，而是躯体、心理与社会行为的完好状态。

因此，谈到健康与疾病预防，教育和医疗应该是其不可分割的两翼。首先是学校的科学教育。科学教育是传播有关疾病预防和卫生健康知识的有效途径。但今天我在这里将集中讨论帮助困境儿童的整合项目。

所有的困境，不仅仅是躯体侵害、性侵害，甚至是缺乏合宜的教养环境（如忽视、冷漠、过重的学习任务等），都会给孩子带来伤害。基本的机制是这些应激源（stress，也就是俗称的心理压力）会引起人体的应激反应，使 HPA 轴（下丘脑—脑垂体—肾上腺轴）产生皮质激素。各种侵害对儿童发展所造成的损害，关键是对 HPA 轴应激反应造成了持久的损害。

为了保护自己，人在进化过程中保留和发展了对外界刺激做出反应的能力。外界具有威胁性的刺激经过感官系统传入大脑，经由下丘脑分别传至不同的脑区，会立即激活一系列身体的生理反应，包括自动激活的交感神经系统、内分泌系统、代谢系统和免疫系统等。其中，HPA 轴是关键。面对威胁，HPA 轴会立即被激活，人体通过下丘脑（H）—脑垂体（P）—肾上腺（A）的路径随即对刺激做出反应。下丘脑释放出 CRH（促肾上腺皮质激素释放激素），刺激脑垂体分泌出 ACTH（促肾上腺皮质激素），ACTH 又刺激肾上腺的外周（即肾上腺皮质）分泌出糖皮质激素。糖皮质激素进入血液循环系统，快速改变人体的植物神经系统和激素系统，提升血糖含量以便为战斗和/或逃逸提供更多的能量，并进一步调整身体的状态，如心跳、呼吸、肌肉收缩力等，以应对外部威胁。

HPA 轴应激反应的特性和糖皮质激素调控 ACTH 和 CRH 的能力与相关脑区的激活状态有关。在应激状态下，HPA 轴被激活。一旦应激源消退，应激系统不同层次上的反馈回路就会被激活，以关闭 HPA 轴的应激反应，使机体恢复到原来的平衡状态。这种调控功能部分是通过与两类受体的结合过程来实现的。这两类受体主要是糖皮质激素受体（GR）和盐皮质激素受体（MR）。这些受体会和到来的皮质激素分子产生特定的结合，并在结合以后启动一系列基因水平的过程，调控许多不同基因的表达。这实际上是表观基因学研究的内容。GR 和 MR 不仅存在于 HPA 轴系统中，也存在于海马区和额叶皮层等脑区。GR 几乎在全身所有的细胞中都会被表达，这就是皮质激素水平的变化会影响很多器官的原因。海马区和额叶皮层两个脑区是调控 HPA 轴恢复平衡态，实现负反馈的重要脑区。另一个脑区是杏仁体，它被称为情绪的发动机。杏仁体会起到与海马区相反的正反馈的作用——激活和加重应激反应。当应激源消退后，额叶皮层会调控杏仁体，让它恢复到原有的平衡状态。

所以，HPA 轴之所以会在进化过程中被保留下来，是因为它具有正面的、有利于人类种族存活的作用。但是如果应激反应过度、持续时间过长，就会产生有害的后果。

按照应激反应产生的影响，可以将应激反应分为以下三类。

（1）正效应的应激反应（positive stress response）。这是正常的生理反应，有时还是促进儿童发展所需要的。例如孩子第一次见到新保姆、学习过程中情绪的存在以及接受预防接种时等，都会产生这一类的应激反应。学习过程中伴有积极的情绪，有利于增强记忆。正效应应激反应的主要特点是会影响心跳，使心跳加速，并会略微增加皮质激素的分泌。在应激源消失后，身体就会回到原有的动态平衡状态。

（2）在容限范围内的应激反应（tolerable stress response）。当人们面对巨大的刺激和打击时，如遭受突如其来的袭击、遇到危险的野兽、遭遇自然灾害、失去亲人等情况下，都会产生应激反应。如果这类应激源存在的时间比较短，特别是有养育者在孩子身边起到支持和缓冲作用，帮助他/她去适应这种冲击，这时机体仍然处于可恢复的弹性状态，在应激源消失后，大脑和身体的其他器官就能从受到伤害的状态中恢复。

（3）有毒害的应激反应（toxic stress response）。如果儿童遭受严重的、频繁的或持续时间长的伤害，且缺乏养育者的必要支持，就会使 HPA 轴持续地处于应激反应状态，这使皮质激素的浓度始终处于不正常的高浓度状态，从而改变 GR 和 MR 的基因表达，降低机体恢复平衡态的调控能力，改变 HPA 轴的响应阈值。同时，高浓度的皮质激素随着血液流经全身，会损坏大脑的结构，影响许多脏器的正常功能。

海马区在学习过程中起着非常重要的作用，它是陈述性记忆形成的部位，直接影响到智力的发展。在身体产生应激反应时，它会起到判别应激源的性质，使 HPA 轴恢复到原有平衡态的负反馈作用。在有毒害的应激反应状态下，皮质激素会损害海马区中神经细胞的功能，削弱使 HPA 轴恢复到原有平衡状态的能力，同时也会降低儿童的记忆力和学习能力。对于一些孕期和早期有困境遭遇的儿童，其海马体的体积会较正常生长的儿童小。类似地，同样负责产生负反馈，控制应激反应，使躯体和大脑恢复到平衡状态的额叶皮层也会发育受阻。此外，前额皮层与杏仁体之间的联系也会减弱，导致情绪调控能力减弱。相反地，有毒害的应激反应会使负责产生刺激反应的杏仁体体积增大，对外来的刺激更加敏感。因此，持续高浓度的皮质激素会降低机体调控 HPA 轴恢复到平衡状态的系统能力，提高 HPA 轴的响应阈值，削弱人对认知和情绪过程的控制。

孕期和儿童早期都是 HPA 轴可塑性最好的时期。在孕期中，无论是因为母亲患有抑郁、焦虑等精神疾病，还是母亲有滥用药品、药物使用不当的情况，如果其经受了有毒害的应激反应，都会对胎儿产生影响。出生以后，在早期的发展过程中，儿童本身产生有毒害的应激反应就会造成进一步的伤害，不仅会影响发育，还会影响到他/她一生的健康和行为，增加其对应激反应相关疾病的易感性，产生认知障碍、增加患精神疾病的风险，发生药物滥用、自杀、暴力等不端行为。Nelson 等对罗马尼亚孤儿院儿童的实证研究也证实了上述机制。

近年来，科学家们还研究了肠道微生物和大脑之间的相互影响，在很大程度上也是通过 HPA 轴产生作用的。

根据科学研究提供的实证，世界卫生组织、联合国儿童基金会和世界银行等国际组织一直在大力呼吁，各国政府和有关方面应该认识到人类可持续发展的根本所在是人类自身的发展，需要认真审视如何能有效地消除贫困和社会经济不平等问题。他们还号召各国将科学研究成果付诸实践，开展整合的救助项目，将贫困地区儿童营养改善项目和儿童早期发展促进项目整合实施。

总之：① 科学研究告诉我们，从受孕到出生后 2~3 年之间的 1000 天，是人类发展的重要时期，既是促进终身发展的机遇期，也是不利条件（贫困、侵害、忽视等）对儿童产生严重不良影响的敏感期。② 早期经受的困境会实质性地嵌入儿童的生物系统，并且改变他们的生物基础和发展过程；会影响这些儿童一生的健康状况，降低他们的认知能力，削弱他们的自我控制能力和情绪控制能力，容易形成上瘾行为、自杀和发展为各类反社会行为。③ 对他们本身造成的这些危害，还可能通过他们成为父母以后的行为传递以及不同的表观基因遗传机制传递给他们的后代。④ 避免和弥补这些不良影响的最有效方法是为这些困境儿童提供持续的、支持性的家庭教养环境。

因此，建议将国家扶贫关注的时间点前移到生命早期的 1000 天，整合医疗、教育和各方面的扶贫力量，支持和改善困境儿童的家庭教养质量，实施帮助困境儿童的整合行动。这是提高精准扶贫、实现教育公平、阻断贫困代际传递的有效措施，这是一项事关中华民族可持续发展的大事。

所有的教育应该遵循教育的规律。教育就是在建构孩子的大脑，所以必须遵循大脑发展的规律，使我们的孩子成为健康的、优秀的社会主义建设者与接班人。顺应发展规律的教育与信息技术的深度融合是教育现代化的重要标志。

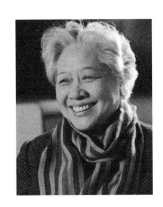

韦钰 中国工程院院士,中国国家教育咨询委员会委员,中国认知科学学会副理事长,MBE 杂志编委,IAP-IBSE 理事会成员。曾任东南大学校长、教育部副部长、中国科协副主席等。

营养助力健康中国

陈君石

国家食品安全风险评估中心

今天我想重点给大家介绍《国民营养计划（2017—2030 年）》，但并不想花太多时间讲内容，因为这个文件网上可以下载到。重点想跟大家介绍一下背景——为什么出台《国民营养计划（2017—2030 年）》以及为什么由国务院来发布。

2012 年，世界卫生组织（WHO）颁布了"2025 年全球营养目标"。2014 年，在罗马召开了第二届国际营养大会，这并不是一般的学术交流，而是政府间的会议。大会由世界卫生组织和联合国粮食及农业组织（FAO）联合举办，150 个国家的代表团参加。此次会议第一次在国际上界定了什么叫作营养不良。在中国，经常说"我们现在面临营养不足和营养过剩的双重负担"，根据罗马会议的界定，这种说法不够科学、不够确切。营养不良的概念包括以下三类问题：

一是营养不足，通俗讲是"吃不饱"，用营养学的专业术语来讲，是蛋白质能量缺乏；

二是微量营养素缺乏，现在比较流行的名词叫作"隐性饥饿"，意思是看起来吃饱了，但是维生素和矿物质摄入不足，所以叫微量营养素缺乏；

三是超重和肥胖，这个界定与传统观念相比有重大改变，而且规范了很多不一致的说法。目前将超重和肥胖统一归为三大类营养不良中的一类，按照中国俗话讲就是"吃动不平衡"。

对照"营养不良"的概念，中国人当前的状况和存在的问题如下。

第一，我们基本上解决了温饱问题，所以我们是基本上吃饱了。当然也存在很少数吃不饱的人，但是从全国 13 亿人口来讲基本上吃饱了。调查数据显示，从 1982 年以来，膳食能量的摄入一直比较充足，人均能量摄入达到甚至超过推荐摄入量。

第二，儿童和少年生长迟缓。我们可以看到，2012 年全国生长迟缓率为 4.7%，几十年来有很大的改善。但是就"农村义务教育学生营养改善计划"的调研结果来看,一些贫困地区与全国平均相比还是有差距的,这些地区 2013 年、2014 年的生长迟缓率分别是 8.0% 和 7.5%。

第三,重要的营养不良问题在于微量营养素的缺乏,首要的是由铁缺乏引起的缺铁性贫血。尽管从总人群来看最近 20 年来贫血率下降非常明显,但是就重点人群分析的话,有 3 个人群贫血率依然较高:特别是 12~24 个月的幼儿以及孕妇,贫血率都在 16% 左右;75 岁及以上高龄老年人的贫血问题也很严重,比儿童、孕妇的贫血率更高一些。

第四,超重和肥胖是我国存在的一个很大的营养问题。刚才王陇德院士在报告中讲的很多慢性病,其共同的主要危险因素就是超重和肥胖。

在这样的背景下,2016—2017 年我们迎来了营养与健康领域最好的政策时代。要解决这些营养问题,政府要出台政策,不仅要考虑中国的政策,更要参考国际政策。目前,联合国可持续发展目标(SDGs)是最大的国际政策性文件。其中目标 2 讲的就是营养:"要消除各种营养不良",同时目标 3 讲的是妇女儿童的健康、传染病、慢性非传染性疾病和紧急事件。要实现以上目标,营养都是重要措施。通俗来讲,营养好了,目标 3 就比较容易实现,营养不好,就很不容易实现或不能实现。

17 个可持续发展目标的内容非常多,除了目标 2 和 3,营养是实现所有其他目标的助推器,即营养能够促使所有目标的完成。总而言之,SDGs 对营养方面的愿景是消除所有形式的营养不良,满足包括生命早期 1000 天在内的整个生命全周期的营养需要,并开展必要的全球营养行动,以获得安全、健康、可持续的食物。

2014 年,习近平总书记提出"没有全民健康,就没有全面小康"。2016 年的"十三五"规划中明确指出"推进健康中国建设",同年 8 月召开了全国卫生与健康大会,同年 10 月发布《"健康中国 2030"规划纲要》(以下简称《规划纲要》)。

《规划纲要》是中央发布的纲领性政策文件,我想强调的是,如果营养没有改善,其中的绝大部分指标肯定是完不成的。因此,营养的重要性是显而易见的。而且《规划纲要》中专门有一节叫作"引导合理膳食",该节第一句话的前半句就是"制定和实施国民营养计划"。在《规划纲要》公布之时,制定国民营养计划的工作已经在进行中。刘延东副总理高瞻远瞩地指示国家卫生计生委牵头起草国民营养计划,那个时候叫"国民营养改善行动计划"。刘延东副总理的指示非常简短,只有两个关键词:一是要与疾病防治相结合,显而易见指的主要是慢性病;二是要拉动食品产业的发展。

国民营养计划的起草工作从 2016 年 2 月启动,到 2017 年 7 月 13 日国务院发布,仅用一年半的时间,效率相当高。作为经历了全过程的专家之一,我深深体会到国务院对国民营养计划的重视。计划的起草由国家卫生计生委牵头，并且多次征求了其他十几个部委的意见。与往常的部门之间文件征求意见所不同的是，这次的征求意见反馈得特别快，而且大家都很有积极性。教育部、农业部等都提出了很好的建议，所以才能够一年半就发布。对于国家卫生计生委上报的草案，国务院不是简单的批准，同时对草案做了非常到位的关键性的修改，并且在出台后马上召开了新闻发布会，充分显示了对其的重视。

《国民营养计划（2017—2030年）》的核心内容有四部分：总体要求、指导思想、基本原则、主要目标。

其中，基本原则有几个亮点：一是坚持科学发展，要充分发挥科技的引领作用；二是坚持创新，促进营养健康与产业融合。注意，是融合，而不是结合，这与刘延东副总理在计划起草之前的指示——"拉动食品产业发展"是非常一致的，所以在后面的很多具体内容都体现了食品产业的发展。

《国民营养计划（2017—2030年）》的主要目标分2020年和2030年两部分，与《"健康中国2030"规划纲要》中的一些健康方面的指标保持一致，并且更细化，如孕妇的叶酸缺乏、中小学生生长迟缓与肥胖并存的问题等。关于肥胖的问题，以学生为目标人群，在起草过程中多次讨论是否提出量化目标。最后讨论的结果是，大家一致认为应实事求是，只要求遏制增长，而不提出具体的百分数。因为，估计到2020年不可能实现学生肥胖率的下降，最好的结果是尽最大努力使上升趋势减缓，因而不定具体量化指标。所以，在计划起草过程中的指标设置和目标设置方面都体现了实事求是的精神。

《国民营养计划（2017—2030年）》的主要内容是告诉人们到底怎么干，国民营养如何改善，体现在以下七项实施策略中。

第一，完善营养法规政策标准体系。几乎所有的发达国家和某一些发展中国家都有国家级营养立法，而中国没有，希望通过《国民营养计划（2017—2030年）》的实施能够突破这一关。

第二，加强营养能力建设。没有足够的能力，所有的目标是不能够完成的。

第三，强化营养和食品安全监测与评估。

第四，发展具有中国特色的食物营养健康产业。这是作为实施策略之一单独提出来的有关食物和食品营养健康产业的内容。

第五，大力发展传统食养服务。

第六，加强营养健康基础数据的共享和利用。全国性的调查研究积累了大量的数据，"如何统一建立数据库实现共享"作为实施策略之一被提出来有很大的指导性意义。

第七，最后一个策略，也是非常重要的策略，即普及营养健康知识。营养能不能改善，关键是要改变人们的行为。人们的行为取决于自身的知识，没有知识不可能改变的。

以上七项实施策略主要针对一般人群，而接下来的主要内容则是六项重大行动，是针对特殊人群的。

第一，生命早期1000天营养健康行动。这是窗口期，所谓窗口期就是在生命早期1000天之内改善营养状况。当然，这不仅仅是营养问题，但如果在这1000天内营养得到改善，人们将会终身受益。换句话说，假如在这1000天内营养不足，就会出现出生后的追赶生长现象，导致成年后超重肥胖、其他各种慢性病及精神病等的高发。这已得到国内外科学研究的证实。

第二，学生营养改善行动。学生也是一个非常重要的特殊人群。

第三，老年人群营养改善行动。现在中国是未富先老，国家还没有真正富裕起来，但是已经进入老龄化社会。根据世界卫生组织的定义，中国现在已经有2亿多老年人，到2030年，这个数字还将继续增加。而老年人的问题比较复杂，营养问题、疾病和养老模式等互相之间都密切相关，所以老年人群的营养改善行动非常必要。

第四，临床营养行动。这点也非常重要。一个简单的例子，假如比较住院患者入院时和出院时的体重，大部分患者出院时体重是下降的。也就是说患者在住院期间的营养没有得到很好的改善，虽然他的疾病治好了或者得到了缓解。这是由于医院对临床营养的重视不够，涉及法律法规的问题、舆论问题、院长们的重视问题以及其他各种各样的问题。与发达国家相比，临床营养师的地位在中国大陆要差很多，甚至与我国台湾地区、香港地区的差距都很大。所以要大力改善临床营养，一定要采取营养评价和营养选择等一系列有针对性的措施，以改善患者的营养状况。

第五，贫困地区营养干预行动。这里强调的是营养干预，因为因病致贫的实际例子很多。起初专家起草时打算将这一行动放在第一位，而国务院把它调到后面的理由也很明确，因为我国到了2020年将会全部脱贫。从政策意义上这很重要，不能说排在后面就不重要了。其实我们很清楚，假如2020年以后不再继续关注这些地区人们的营养状况，那贫困的帽子还会戴回去。

第六，吃动平衡行动。饮食很重要，但体育锻炼也不能被忽视。

除了以上六项重大行动，最后一个重要部分是加强组织实施。有几点意义重大，例如各级地方政府要通过纳入政府绩效考核来强化组织保障。认真实施《国民营养计划（2017—2030年）》并不是一句空话。首先要保障经费投入，加大对国民营养计划的投入力度。营养问题不能仅靠政府投入，更要充分依托各方面的资金渠道。其次，我们还必须加强国际合作、强化组织领导、广泛宣传动员。

最后，简要小结一下。营养学是现代医学的一部分，也是现代预防医学的一部分，与国人的健康和疾病息息相关。实施《"健康中国 2030"规划纲要》，全面建成小康社会，离不开营养学，或者更大众化的说法是离不开老百姓营养状况的改善。目前，中国人基本上解决了温饱问题，但是还存在微量营养素的缺乏（如前面提到的铁缺乏，还有锌缺乏、碘缺乏等问题也存在，以及钙、维生素 A、维生素 D 等一系列微量营养素缺乏）、超重和肥胖等问题。因此，还有很多问题有待我们解决。

《国民营养计划（2017—2030 年）》的正式发布，特别是作为国务院文件发布，将对全方位推动营养工作，实现全面小康，助力健康中国的梦想起到重要的作用。

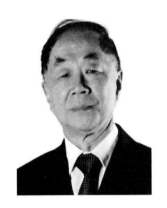

陈君石　中国工程院院士，国家食品安全风险评估中心总顾问，国家食品安全风险评估专家委员会主任委员，国家食品安全标准审评委员会副主任委员，国务院食品安全委员会专家委员会副主任，中华预防医学会健康风险评估与控制专业委员会主任委员，世界卫生组织食品安全专家团成员，国际生命科学学会中国办事处主任。

中国心血管病的现状和防治策略

高润霖

国家心血管病中心,中国医学科学院阜外医院

目前心血管病已经成为我国城乡居民第一位的死亡原因,按照国家卫生计生委最新的统计数据,农村心血管病死亡率占 45%,城市心血管病死亡率占 42%。农村心血管病死亡率已经超过了城市。我国面临的心血管病疾病负担十分沉重。

一、中国心血管病现状

据《中国心血管病报告 2014》估计,我国现有心血管病患者 2.9 亿,其中高血压患病人数 2.7 亿、脑卒中 700 万、心肌梗死 250 万、心衰 450 万。而且发病率、死亡率还在不断增加。从 1990 年到 2015 年,中国城乡居民心血管病死亡率一直在升高,农村升高得更快,且已经超过了城市(图 1)。

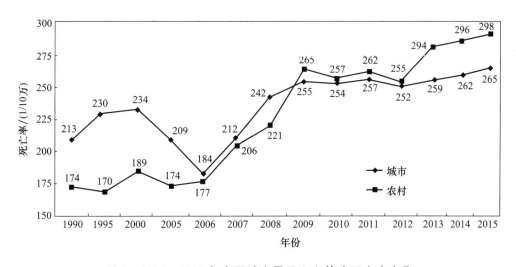

图 1　1990—2015 年中国城乡居民心血管病死亡率变化

(引自《中国心血管病报告 2016》)

心血管病包括冠心病和脑血管病。脑血管病近年来死亡率增长的趋势变缓,城市脑血管病死亡率已经基本上趋于平缓,农村仍在升高且已高于城市。按年龄

标化的死亡率变化分析，心血管病的标化死亡率仍然在增加，男性增加明显。但1990 年到 2013 年脑卒中的标化死亡率已经降低（图 2），表明我国在脑卒中防治方面已经取得了初步成绩。然而，冠心病的标化死亡率依然在上升（图 3），过去城市明显高于农村，现在农村和城市已经基本持平。尤其是急性心肌梗死的死亡率，不论是农村还是城市，都明显增加，而且农村增速明显快于城市。为什么会出现这样的情况呢？主要由于人们生活方式的改变、危险因素的流行，农村发病增速快，但防控措施未能跟上，治疗条件较城市差，病死率高，造成农村心肌梗死的死亡率高于城市。据 China-PEACE 的研究，2001—2011 年 10 年间我国心肌梗死住院数增加近 5 倍，但心肌梗死住院病死率无明显变化。改善心肌梗死预后的最重要治疗方法是再灌注治疗（急诊介入治疗或溶栓）。然而，这 10 年中再灌注治疗的比例基本没有变化。急诊介入治疗的比例有所增加，但溶栓的比例相应减少，导致再灌注治疗的比例在 10 年中没有明显变化，这也是急性心肌梗死住院死亡率没有降低的主要原因。根据 CAMI 注册研究，近年来我国各级医院再灌注治疗的比例有所增加，其中省级以上医院再灌注治疗比例明显增加，高于市级、县级医院，省级医院的住院病死率明显低于县级医院。

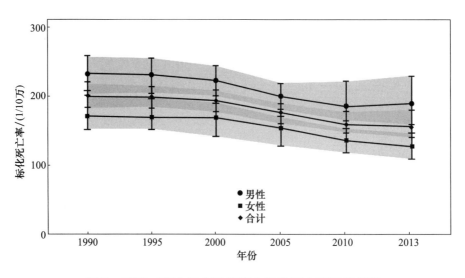

图 2　1990—2013 年中国脑卒中标化死亡率变化趋势

（ZHOU M,et al. Lancet. 2016,387:251-272.）

2001 年到 2011 年，我国心血管病住院人数增加了 5 倍，住院经济负担显著增加。与发达国家相比，我国心血管防治任重道远。例如脑卒中的发生，日本曾经是脑卒中的"大国"，但经过多年的防治，其脑卒中死亡人数大幅降低。目前，中国脑卒中死亡率是日本的 4 倍，也是美国的 4 倍，这说明我国的防控任务非常艰巨。

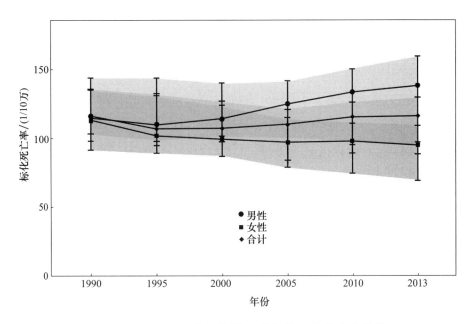

图 3 1990—2013 年中国冠心病标化死亡率变化趋势

（ZHOU M,et al. Lancet. 2016,387:251-272.）

按照"中国冠心病预测模型"预测:2010 年到 2030 年,如果仅考虑人口老龄化和人口增长因素,35 岁到 84 岁人群中心血管病患者数量将增加 50%,如果考虑高血压、胆固醇、糖尿病、吸烟等因素,心血管病患者数量将额外增加 23%。

二、中国老龄化及心血管病的危险因素

心血管病主要是由年龄和心血管病的危险因素造成的。城镇化、老龄化是不可避免的。从 2005 年我国就已经进入了老龄化社会。按 65 岁以上人口计算,我国老年人口 2005 年是 1 亿,到 2017 年是 1.4 亿;60 岁以上人口已经达到 2 亿。

心血管病的危险因素主要包括高血压、高胆固醇、肥胖、水果蔬菜摄入不足、吸烟、饮酒、糖尿病等,其中高血压和高胆固醇这两个危险因素最重要。发达国家胆固醇的贡献率比高血压高,发展中国家(包括中国)高血压的贡献率更高,但胆固醇的贡献率也不容忽视。

现在我国心血管病危险因素的变化情况如何呢? 根据 MUCA 的研究,我国 80% 以上的心血管病(包括冠心病和缺血性脑卒中)可归因于主要危险因素,其中 35% 归因于高血压、32% 归因于吸烟、11% 归因于高胆固醇血症、3% 归因于糖尿病。最重要的危险因素——高血压的患病率在不断上升。1959 年,18 岁以上人口患病率为 5.1%,1991 年为 12.6%,2002 年为 18.8%,我国"十二五"期间心血管病患病率调查项目抽样调查了 50 万人群,高血压的粗患病率为 28%,加权患病率为 23.2%。我国高血压的患病率一路走高,且随着年龄的增长呈上升趋势,50 岁

以上人群患病率为 50% 以上,70 岁以上人群患病率达 60% 以上。近年来,高血压的防治取得了一定的成效。根据 2015 年调查,高血压知晓率为 51.5%、治疗率为 46.1%、控制率为 16.9%;而 1991 年知晓率仅为 26%、治疗率为 12%、控制率为 3%。虽然,"三率"水平与发达国家相比仍有较大差距,但应该说高血压的防治在国家大力安排组织之下还是取得了一定的进步。由于脑卒中与高血压的关系更大,近年来我国脑卒中标化死亡率的降低至少部分与高血压的防治有关。

胆固醇是冠心病最重要的危险因素。北京地区 1984—1999 年冠心病的死亡人数增加,77% 归因于胆固醇的升高。1984 年到 1999 年,北京居民平均胆固醇水平上升了 24%。2012 年血脂调查结果显示,低密度脂蛋白胆固醇升高超过 130 mg/dL 的人数占 20.4%。如果不严格控制胆固醇升高的话,冠心病的发病率会进一步增加。目前,我国高胆固醇血症的患病率呈上升趋势,对高胆固醇血症的控制较差。根据 PURE 对 17 个国家社区医院的调查,我国冠心病二级预防使用他汀类药物者仅有 2%,远远低于欧美国家,仅比非洲(1.4%)多一点。当然,这只是 PURE 研究的抽样调查,样本不一定具有代表性。但这至少可以说明,我国对他汀类药物用于冠心病二级预防与临床需要之间仍有较大差距。随着胆固醇升高与冠心病发病率的关系越来越密切,我国冠心病标化死亡率仍在上升的事实,就不难理解了。

糖尿病也是心血管病的一个重要危险因素。我国成人糖尿病患病率达 9.7%。此外,吸烟也是我国心血管病的一个重要危险因素。近年来,经过大力开展控烟运动,减少的比例非常有限,控烟工作还远远不够。超重肥胖人数也在增加。

三、心血管病防治措施

(一)预防为主,控制危险因素

人口老龄化的趋势是不可阻挡的,也是我们不能改变的,但危险因素是可以改变的。一系列研究表明,如果控制了危险因素,就可以减少 78%~89% 的冠心病发病、78%~85% 的冠心病死亡、70%~76% 的脑卒中发病、65%~73% 的脑卒中死亡。所以,要防治心脑血管病,必须把战线前移,从控制危险因素入手,以预防为主。正所谓"上医医未病之病"。

国际上已有许多控制危险因素降低心血管病死亡的成功范例。1968 年到 1981 年,美国心血管病死亡率的降低远较非心血管病死亡率的降低更明显。第二次世界大战后,美国人由于生活水平明显提高,胆固醇摄入明显增加,高血压患者增多,心血管病死亡人数呈爆发式增长。但由于国家胆固醇教育计划以及高血压防治计划的实施,其心血管病的死亡率明显下降。现在美国冠心病死亡率下降了30%以上,脑卒中死亡率下降了近50%。研究表明,美国心血管病死亡率的降低,65%归因于改善危险因素,其中24%归因于降低胆固醇、20%归因于人群血压下降。根据美国的经验,有效防控危险因素特别是控制高血压和降低胆固醇是降低心血管病死亡率的最重要措施。芬兰曾经是世界上心血管病死亡率最高的国家之一。芬兰通过北卡(North Carolina)计划的研究和实施,通过控烟和改变生活习惯,减少奶油摄入量,使北卡地区心血管病死亡率降低了80%之多,而芬兰全国心血管病死亡率下降了50%。芬兰的经验也非常值得我们借鉴。

我国也有心血管预防研究的成功经验。大庆研究在20世纪80年代开始对糖尿病前期患者进行生活方式干预,干预一年后,随访23年累积全因死亡率较对照组降低29%。经验表明,通过群防群治,控制高血压,可显著降低脑卒中的发病率和死亡率。

1979年,英国著名流行病学家Geoffrey Rose首先提出预防心血管病的两种策略,即全人群策略和高危人群策略。美国疾病控制与预防中心(CDC)的报告认为,让公众获得心血管病防治知识,是降低心血管病发病率最根本的治疗措施,也是最经济的治疗手段。通过改变生活方式,使美国人的高血压发病率减少了55%、脑卒中发病率减少了75%、糖尿病发病率减少了50%、癌症发病率减少了1/3、国民的预期寿命增加10年。

(二)政府主导,"把健康融入所有政策"

预防控制心脑血管病,一定要由政府主导。习近平主席在全国卫生与健康大会上强调,把人民健康放在优先发展的战略地位,将健康融入所有政策。习主席指出,要坚定不移地贯彻预防为主方针,坚持防治结合、联防联控、群防群控,努力为人民群众提供全生命周期的卫生与健康服务。习主席的重要指示也为心血管病防治指明了方向。

心血管病作为最常见的慢性病,其防治工作必须由政府主导,将防治关口前移,以预防为主,这样才能有效地控制心血管病的发生。

(三)加强分级诊疗制度建设

为了有效防控心血管病,加强分级诊疗制度建设十分重要。我国现在大约有2.9亿心血管病患者,其中至少有2.7亿高血压人群。如前所述,高血压是最重要的心血管病危险因素,如果高血压患者中50%就诊于三级医院,那么每个医院每天要接诊 320 个高血压患者,医院不堪重负,医生没有时间与患者充分交流,更不能做到随访。采取分级诊疗可有效解决这个问题。强调基层首诊,加强联动。大部分患者在社区就诊,社区医疗机构可以及早发现高血压患者,对一般高血压患者给予治疗,并进行随访,观察治疗效果。如果血压控制得不好,可以转到二级医院,按指南调整药物。二级医院可将难处理的患者转到三级医院和专科医院进行进一步检查,调整治疗,必要时做进一步检查排除继发性高血压。血压稳定后再转回二级医院、社区医疗机构,长期随访,观察疗效。这样就形成了一个有效的高血压防治体系。社区进行预防高血压的健康宣教,定期检查,早期发现高血压患者,提高高血压的知晓率、治疗率和控制率,使高血压得到有效控制,从而有效降低脑卒中、冠心病的发病率和死亡率。

高血压作为慢性病,其分级诊疗是从下往上的;而急性心肌梗死是一种死亡率较高的急性疾病,其分级诊疗应该是从上而下。急性胸痛疑似心肌梗死的患者应立即呼叫救护车,在救护车上就开始联系医院,把患者送到有急诊介入治疗(PCI)条件的医院,通过绿色通道尽快进行急诊 PCI。如果患者被送到无 PCI 条件的医院,应尽快进行溶栓治疗,然后转至上级医院进行冠脉造影,必要时进行PCI。患者病情稳定后,可转到二级医院进行康复治疗。这样才能提高再灌注治疗的比例,缩短首次医疗接触至再灌注治疗的时间,降低急性心肌梗死的死亡率。

(四) 慢性病规范化管理落地

另外一个问题,要规范慢性病的管理,而且规范一定要落地。首先应该制定慢性病管理规范、指南、临床路径。高血压、糖尿病健康管理现已被列为国家财政拨款且覆盖全部居民的国家基本公共卫生服务项目。最近公布的一项调查显示,在 3362 个基层医疗单位中,8.1% 的医院根本没有降压药,只有 33.8% 的单位有四种经循证医学证实有效的降压药。如果药都没有,何谈高血压控制?因此政策落地非常重要。

(五) 推动"医疗保障"向"健康保障"转型

最后一点,是关于医疗保障的问题,我们应该推动医疗保障向健康保障转型。现在我们的医保主要还是保障治疗,消耗巨大。比如现在冠心病的标化死亡率在增高,这些晚期患者要花掉大量医保资金,如果从上游控制高胆固醇血症的话,冠心病发病率可以减少 20%。但高胆固醇血症没有症状,如不化验,不能发现,患者知晓率非常低。通常发现以后也没得到适当的治疗。如果胆固醇升高这个重要危险因素不能控制,冠心病怎么能得到控制呢?所以我们建议"三高"共管,现在高血压、糖尿病已经纳入基本卫生服务项目,应该把高胆固醇血症也纳入其中,这样才能更有效地控制危险因素,降低心血管病死亡率。这就需要医保部门改变观念,从医疗保障向健康保障转型。

(六)发挥"互联网+"的作用

另外,我们利用互联网技术对患者和公众进行健康宣教、对基层医生进行培训、做远程会诊平台、进行医院联盟医疗指导。"互联网+"将发挥非常重要的作用。

四、结论

心血管病是我国城乡居民第一位的死亡原因,且死亡率仍呈上升趋势。心血管病死亡率上升主要由于人口老龄化和危险因素的流行。高血压、高胆固醇血症、糖尿病、吸烟、超重肥胖等是最重要的危险因素。防治心血管病的关键是防控危险因素,坚持政府主导,以预防为主,规范防治管理落地,建立分级诊疗制度,推动"医疗保障"向"健康保障"转型,充分发挥"互联网+"的作用。我国心血管病死亡率下降的拐点一定能够早日到来。

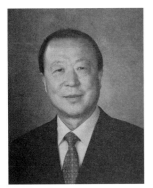

高润霖 中国工程院院士,心血管病学专家。1965 年毕业于北京医科大学,1981 年在中国协和医科大学获硕士学位。曾任中国医学科学院心血管病研究所所长、阜外心血管病医院院长、心内科主任。现任国家心血管病中心专家委员会主任委员,阜外医院心内科首席专家,研究员,博士生导师。

长期工作在临床第一线,从事心血管病临床、科研及人群防治工作,是我国介入心脏病学的先驱者之一。他为介入心脏病学学科建立和发展,为我国冠心病介入治疗的普及、推广、规范化及器材国产化做出了重要贡献。作为主要研究者完成了我国"十二五"科技支撑项目——中国重要心血管病患病率调查及关键技术研究。

健康中国——呼吸系统疾病早诊早治战略

钟南山

广州医科大学,国家呼吸系统疾病临床医学研究中心

当今,呼吸系统疾病严重威胁我国人民的健康。在中国,影响呼吸系统的主要因素包括严重的空气污染、吸烟和频发重大急性呼吸系统传染病。慢性病死亡人数占我国总死亡人数的 87%,慢性呼吸系统疾病占 11%[1],严重威胁国民健康。呼吸系统疾病防控是健康中国战略的重大需求。我国临床防治战略的发展方向应从"4P"模式,即预测性(predictive)、预防性(preventive)、个体化(personalized)和参与性(participatory),转向"5P"模式,即在"4P"模式基础上加上早干预(presymptomatic)。

吸烟是导致呼吸系统疾病的危险因素。美国加州最初烟草消费比其他州高,但随着控烟政策的实施,其烟草消费水平出现下降。通过 40 年控烟政策的支持,加州的烟草消费量相较于其他州出现了显著下降[2]。1960—2007 年,经过近 50 年的发展,相较于美国、英国和日本明显下降的趋势,中国的吸烟率仍保持在较高水平,如图 1 所示。

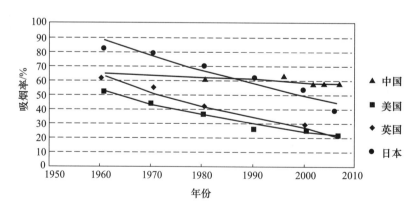

图 1　部分国家男性吸烟率变化趋势

除了吸烟问题,空气污染问题也是我国呼吸系统疾病高发的不可忽视的一个重要诱因。在 2012—2015 年期间,通过在广东省选取 4 个地区(广州与湛江分别代表城区,韶关和河源分别代表农村地区),其中分别随机抽取 2 个街道或者村庄,将区域内 20 岁以上人群纳入研究的方法进行了一项空气污染与慢阻肺关系的研究。研究显示,慢阻肺的患病率与 PM 浓度显著相关[3]:当 PM2.5 由 35 mg/m³ 升至 75 mg/m³,慢阻肺患病危险增加 2.416 倍;当 PM10 由 50 mg/m³ 升至 150 mg/m³,慢阻肺患病危险增加 2.442 倍。这意味着 PM 2.5 每增加 10 mg/m³,FEV1(第一秒用力呼气量)下降 25 mL。由此可见,空气污染对呼吸系统造成了极大的威胁。

另外,应提高早期肺癌的诊断率,降低肺癌总死亡率,从而实现早期诊断、早期干预。肺癌随疾病发展分期越晚,5 年存活率越低[4]。因此,肺癌的早期筛查对于早防早治有重要的意义。在广州市人民政府、广州市卫生计生委、广州市民政局的支持下,以广州医科大学附属第一医院及国家呼吸系统疾病临床医学研究中心为依托,在社区网络的协助下,先后开展了低保低收入人群及越秀区居民的免费肺癌筛查项目,为符合条件的居民提供免费的低剂量螺旋 CT 及肿瘤标志物检测,目的是提高早期肺癌的诊断率,从而降低肺癌总死亡率。除了早期筛查,广州呼吸疾病研究所胸外科团队还针对早期肺癌术后复发的临床问题分析了与复发相关的临床特征,基于临床因素的列线图筛选出肿瘤的相关基因,通过 L2 COX等比风险统计法建立了多基因表达预测模型,并在国际上发表了这两个生存预测模型[5-6],这在一定意义上可以作为一种改善肺癌预后的临床预测方法。

2015 年,全球有约 320 万人死于慢阻肺(COPD),较 1990 年增加了11.6%[7]。慢阻肺长期维持治疗策略首先应关注早期病变,因为慢阻肺患者早期阶段占比最高(即 GOLD I-II 级)。在美国,GOLD Ⅰ-Ⅱ级患者占所有慢阻肺患者的 76%[8],在中国也几乎占据了 70.7%[9]。*GOLD 2006*(《全球 COPD 防治指南 2006》)将GOLD 0 级的定义取消,其原因是缺乏足够证据支持 GOLD 0 级的患者将发展为GOLD Ⅰ 级[10]。但最近的资料表明,在生活质量和活动能力方面,GOLD 0 级接近于 GOLD Ⅰ 级,而且超过 50% 的 GOLD 0 级人群存在呼吸相关损伤[11]。通过OCT 技术(光学相干断层扫描技术)检测小气道病变,可以发现相当一部分重度吸烟者虽然肺功能正常,但小气道结构已发生改变[12],这可以作为 GOLD 0 级的证据。

慢阻肺患者通常在 FEV1 明显下降时(FEV1≤50%)才出现症状[13]。与健康人相比,所有 GOLD 级别的患者都会出现 FEV1 逐年下降的趋势,Ⅰ-Ⅱ级患者下降更为显著[14-16],即早期慢阻肺患者肺功能下降速率较快。因此,早期慢阻肺特点就是以小气道病变为主,症状轻,常被忽视,远动耐量已有降低,FEV1 年递减率最快。

慢阻肺的治疗战略最重要的是早期诊断、早期治疗。*GOLD 2018*(《全球

COPD 防治指南 2018》)指出,慢阻肺是一种常见的、可以预防和治疗的疾病,其特征是持续存在的呼吸系统症状和气流受限,通常与显著暴露于毒性颗粒与气体引起的气道和/或肺泡异常相关。根据慢阻肺的定义,任何存在呼吸困难、慢性咳嗽或咳痰并伴有/或有危险因素暴露史的患者,都应考虑慢阻肺的诊断。确诊需要通过肺通气功能检测(吸入支气管舒张剂后 FEV1/FVC < 0.70)。在指南中关注的是出现症状后才做出诊断。中国对慢阻肺的诊断和治疗严重不足。在研究中被诊断为慢阻肺的患者中,仅有 35.1% 的患者曾被确诊为慢阻肺,说明慢阻肺的严重诊断不足;病情相对较轻的 II 级患者中,64.7% 的患者至少具有一种呼吸症状,但大部分患者未接受过治疗,说明慢阻肺的治疗不足[9]。

由广州医科大学附属第一医院广州呼吸疾病研究所牵头的 Tie-COPD 研究项目通过对社区慢阻肺患者初筛,选择 GOLD I-II 级(无症状或仅有极少症状)患者入组,进行噻托溴铵两年持续用药,以安慰剂组为对照的随机、双盲、平行分组、多中心临床研究,以第 24 个月时 FEV1 较基线变化的组间差异为研究的主要结果测量指标。研究结果表明,与安慰剂组相比,噻托溴铵持续显著改善患者 FEV1、FVC,且噻托溴铵组的 FEV1 年递减率较安慰剂组低;相较于安慰剂组,噻托溴铵组能显著降低首次急性加重的发生风险,显著延长距首次急性加重时间,显著降低急性加重发生率/住院率,持续改善患者生活质量[17]。Tie-COPD 研究项目是首个噻托溴铵干预早期慢阻肺(GOLD I-II 级)的前瞻性研究。噻托溴铵可持续显著改善肺功能,减缓 FEV1 年递减率(包括 CAT<10,即无明显症状患者),也可改善生活质量,降低急性加重的风险;药物干预早期慢阻肺患者能带来临床收益,为疾病的防治前移提供更多的证据,减轻患者和社会的负担。随访初步显示,两组患者的 FEV1 在停用噻托溴铵一年后未显示差别,说明即使是早期慢阻肺患者也需要持续干预治疗。最新的 COPD 防治指南建议在有症状的患者中寻找慢阻肺病例(case-finding),但并不推荐筛查无症状的人群。美国预防医学服务特别行动委员会(USPSTF)也不推荐在没有症状的成年人中进行慢阻肺的筛查[18]。我不支持这种观点,Tie-COPD 研究推荐在有长期暴露在危险因素(如吸烟、使用生物燃料烹调、暴露于严重大气污染)下的人群中进行筛查(即使无症状);发现早期慢阻肺患者需要持续治疗。类似于高血压、糖尿病的早期干预战略,这也是我们预防医学在慢阻肺诊治中的早期干预新战略。

习近平主席在 2016 年全国卫生与健康大会上提出我国健康与卫生工作的方针:"以基层为重点,以改革创新为动力,预防为主,中西医并重,将健康融入所有政策,人民共建共享"。若不注重早防早治,出现症状后才开始治疗甚至抢救,医疗费用肯定会节节攀升;相反,如果注重早防早治,减少症状出现后才进行治疗或者抢救的机会,医疗费用自然会下降。因此,我国临床防治战略的发展方向应是早期预防、早期干预。

参 考 文 献

[1] WHO. Noncommunicable diseases: country profiles 2014. 2014.

[2] PIERCE J P, MESSER K, WHITE M M, et al. Forty years of faster decline in cigarette smoking in California explains current lower lung cancer rates. Cancer Epidemiology, Biomarkers & Prevention, 2010, 19: 2801-2810.

[3] LIU S, ZHOU Y, LIU S, et al. Association between exposure to ambient particulate matter and chronic obstructive pulmonary disease: results from a cross-sectional study in China. Thorax, 2017, 72: 788-795.

[4] DETTERBECK F C, BOFFA D J, TANOUE LT. The new lung cancer staging system. Chest, 2009, 136: 260-271.

[5] LIANG W, ZHANG L, JIANG G, et al. Development and validation of a nomogram for predicting survival in patients with resected non-small-cell lung cancer. Journal of Clinical Oncology, 2015, 33: 861-869.

[6] KRATZ J R, HE J, VAN DEN EEDEN S K, et al. A practical molecular assay to predict survival in resected non-squamous, non-small-cell lung cancer: development and international validation studies. Lancet, 2012, 379: 823-832.

[7] SORIANO J B, ABAJOBIR A A, ABATE K H, et al. Global, regional, and national deaths, prevalence, disability-adjusted life years, and years lived with disability for chronic obstructive pulmonary disease and asthma, 1990-2015: a systematic analysis for the Global Burden of Disease Study 2015. Lancet Respiratory Medicine, 2017, 5: 691-706.

[8] MAPEL D W, DALAL A A, BLANCHETTE C M, et al. Severity of COPD at initial spirometry-confirmed diagnosis: data from medical charts and administrative claims. International Journal of Chronic Obstructive Pulmonary Disease, 2011, 6: 573-581.

[9] ZHONG N, WANG C, YAO W, et al. Prevalence of chronic obstructive pulmonary disease in China: a large, population-based survey. American Journal of Respiratory and Critical Care Medicine, 2007, 176: 753-760.

[10] VESTBO J, LANGE P. Can GOLD Stage 0 provide information of prognostic value in chronic obstructive pulmonary disease. American Journal of Respiratory and Critical Care Medicine, 2002, 166: 329-332.

[11] REGAN E A, LYNCH D A, CURRAN-EVERETT D, et al. Clinical and radiologic disease in smokers with normal spirometry. JAMA Internal Medicine, 2015, 175: 1539-1549.

[12] DING M, CHEN Y, GUAN W J, et al. Measuring airway remodeling in patients with different COPD staging using endobronchial optical coherence tomography. Chest, 2016, 150: 1281-1290.

[13] SUTHERLAND E R, CHERNIACK R M. Management of chronic obstructive pulmonary disease. The New England Journal of Medicine, 2004, 350: 2689-2697.

[14] WELTE T, VOGELMEIER C, PAPI A. COPD: early diagnosis and treatment to slow disease progression. International Journal of Clinical Practice, 2015, 69: 336-349.

[15] TANTUCCI C, MODINA D. Lung function decline in COPD. International Journal of Chronic Obstructive Pulmonary Disease, 2012, 7: 95-99.

[16] PITTA F, TROOSTERS T, SPRUIT M A, et al. Characteristics of physical activities in daily life in chronic obstructive pulmonary disease. American Journal of Respiratory and Critical Care Medicine, 2005, 171：972-977.

[17] ZHOU Y, ZHONG N S, LI X, et al. Tiotropium in early-stage chronic obstructive pulmonary disease. The New England Journal of Medicine, 2017, 377：923-935.

[18] FORCE USPST, SIU A L, BIBBINS-DOMINGO K, et al. Screening for chronic obstructive pulmonary disease：US preventive services task force recommendation statement. JAMA, 2016, 315：1372-1377.

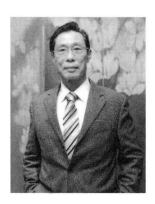

钟南山　中国工程院院士，国家呼吸系统疾病临床医学研究中心主任，广州医科大学呼吸内科教授、博士生导师，"973"首席科学家，中华医学会前会长、顾问。爱丁堡大学荣誉教授，伯明翰大学科学博士（Doctor of Science），英国皇家内科学会高级会员（爱丁堡、伦敦），首届"港大百周年杰出学者"。

卫生政策综合协调的原因和举措

Evelyne de Leeuw

健康公平培训、研究与评价中心（CHETRE）

俗话说,世上只有两件事确定无疑:死亡和纳税。这则比喻用在当前国际视野的卫生政策和改善上再恰当不过。虽然世界人口平均预期寿命正在增长,但寿命的延长存在两个问题。一是生命所延长的时间未必都是高质量时间。世界上大多数国家,人们生命的最后四分之一都是在疾病或非健康状态（尤其是一些所谓非传染慢性疾病的积累）下度过的。对于大多数现在希望活过 80 岁的人来说,他们生命中平均有 16 年将在非健康状态下度过。同时,还有另一因素使这一问题更加尖锐。不同人群所享有的卫生条件有明显的差异和不公平。这种不公平不仅体现在预期寿命（人口健康的一个非常粗略的衡量标准）上,也体现在生活质量和健康状态下的生命长度上。有一个专业术语可以充分揭示这两个问题导致的现象,即"社会梯度"（social gradient）[1]——那些拥有更高社会地位、更体面职业、更可观收入且接受更好教育、享有更好社会保障的人往往享有更好的医疗卫生条件,他们的寿命更长,而且也更为健康。

与世界上大多数预防性卫生政策想要我们相信的情况相反,这同个人生活方式的选择关系并不大。在选择社会地位、体面就业、可观收入、尽可能好的教育、高质量住房、健全的法律支持和安全保障体系等方面,个人所能够选择的空间和潜力非常微渺。

所有这些促进健康条件的因素（也被称为健康的社会、政治和商业决定因素）都取决于集体决策,取决于社会集体（无论是联邦、基督教信徒群体,还是穆斯林架构的社会体系）分配（或再分配）资源的方式。事实上,这的确与税收有关,而且不是所有的税收都是平等的。在一些国家,对非健康产品（比如烟草、酒水和高含糖量饮料）的征税明显提高,用以回馈卫生改善系统。在澳大利亚的联邦层面、韩国的地方政府层面,这种做法都得到了推行。在一些其他国家,非健康产品所征税收用于补贴全民医疗保健系统和其他福利保障（比如探亲假）。然而，在有些国家，这类举措还是缺失的，需要个人去安排。此类分配和再分配政策未必需要现有证据证明其能促进卫生改善和人口繁衍。

我们知道，公共卫生政策介入是我们可以想到的最好的社会投资。传统上，这类投资包括疫苗接种计划和乘车系牢安全带要求。每一个货币单位的投资都带来了更多的收益和回报。但这显然超出了可以被认同的传统卫生领域投资。同样货币单位投资于提高女孩识字率的项目所产生的卫生收益，远远高于其投资于医疗护理领域所带来的卫生收益。

再说说一些众所周知的俗语和箴言。虽然死亡和纳税确定无疑，我们还是更愿意相信"一天一苹果，医生远离我"（an apple a day keeps the doctor away）的俗语。然而，有证据充分表明，政府并没有在践行这一智慧上发挥突出作用。根据荷兰国家公共卫生与环境研究院所做的研究，一小部分公共卫生预算用于疾病预防，而只有很小一部分预算用于健康促进。因此，世界各国均将大量预算花费在了疾病领域，可以说，花费了大量金钱用于解决一些本可以在最初就避免的问题，或者是花费了巨大的成本却未得到就生命质量而言应有的收益。从某种意义上讲，国家的卫生预算是浪费的，而且并没有带来真正的健康。美国拥有世界上最昂贵的医疗保健系统，同时也是世界上医疗卫生最不公平的国家之一，这便是最好不过的例子。

一、什么造就了健康（公平）？

如果各国政府要认真履行其保护和提高人民健康水平的职责并确保社会公平从而保证社会的任何群体不被落下，那么就很有必要了解"什么造就了健康"。这与"什么导致了疾病"这个问题完全不同。针对后者，生物医学界有广泛的论述，从各类病原体（如病毒等）出发，用研究病理学的笛卡尔式思维就可以轻松地回答。但是"什么造就了健康"却是一个完全不同的问题。

在20世纪60年代晚期至70年代早期，Henrik Blum教授是率先思考这一问题的学者之一[2]。Blum曾同就职于加拿大卫生部长期卫生规划司的Hubert Laframboise[3]一起工作过——他在1974年出版的著名政府文件《加拿大人对健康的新视角》的撰写中发挥了重要作用。这份文件也被称作"拉隆德报告"（以首倡这一报告的拉隆德部长命名），该文件首次明确指出，人类的生理状况、生活方式、医疗保健和环境因素共同造就了健康。更加精细的观点明显表明健康不仅仅局限于上述四个领域，而且这四个领域不能完全阐释清楚各健康决定因素之间的动态关系。

后来，另一支加拿大团队[4]承担起这一挑战，他们试图阐释健康的社会梯度。

他们努力探索导致不同群体健康结果差异的路径(图1)。虽然也有生理学路径(他们可能会适应生活方式的改变甚至是药物干预),但关键的发现是社会和环境系统在塑造健康机遇和积极健康状况过程中发挥着非常重要的作用[5]。反过来,这意味着(地方、区域和国家)政府等社会系统甚至是私人工作场所都要为创造并维系健康制定标准和政策。

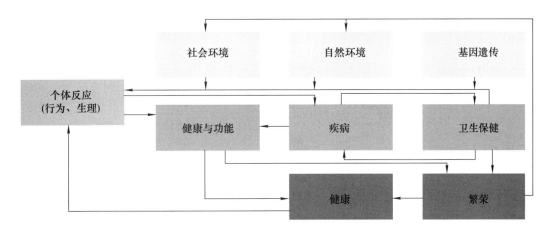

图1 什么导致了不同群体的健康差异[4]

这当然不是最新的发现。基于世界卫生组织 20 世纪 80 年代委任的工作,Dahlgren 和 Whitehead[6]发表了他们被广泛认可的健康与卫生公平的"彩虹"社会模式(图2)。但更早以前,世界上的原住民就已经知道和谐、平衡和社会生态系统是造就与维系健康的必需因素。

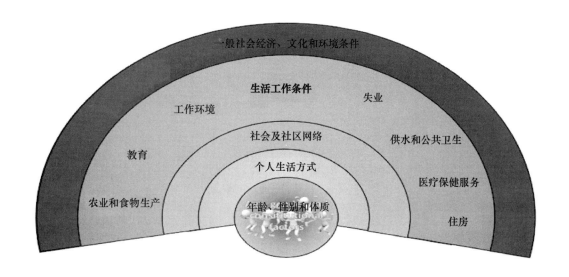

图2 著名的健康决定因素彩虹模型:"逐层影响"[6]

二、我们想要的不是更多问题,而是解决方案

自从健康的社会决定因素的论点问世以来,学术界和政策落实者(非指社会活动价)就开始为解决这一社会和道德不公正问题而困扰[7]。世界卫生组织及其成员国如芬兰、瑞典、丹麦和荷兰都在研究健康的社会决定因素和卫生不公平背后的政策原因[8]。一般来说,同美国、英国和澳大利亚一样,他们一致认为解决这一综合问题需要综合施策。比如,英国政府的咨询文件《处理英格兰的卫生不公平问题》中指出:"《艾奇逊报告》研究了健康决定因素的'逐层影响理论'……解决卫生不公平问题需要我们研究这些'逐层的影响'。"2002 年,威尔士卫生政策指出:"缓解卫生不公平需要一个多方面的综合性战略……从而把握健康的经济和环境决定因素"[8]。

虽然关于健康的社会决定因素和卫生公平的学术理论呈爆炸式增长,但似乎很少有国家(或者地方政府)可以落实这样的洞见,在专业、深刻的分析论证基础上制定系统的、综合的、多维度全方位的解决方案。

显然,各政府部门正在为"逐层影响理论"涉及政府主管的各个领域而困惑,卫生公平的发展和可持续性也客观要求包括卫生部门在内的众多部门都参与进来。

一个被公认的早期政策解决方案来自 1986 年的《健康促进渥太华宪章》(以下简称《宪章》),该宪章首次采用了"建立健康的公共政策"("Healthy Public Policy",这一短语由 Nancy Milio[9]和 Trevor Hancock[10]同时创造)的愿景。在 20世纪 80 年代中期[11],他们意外地创造了这一短语。Milio 继续创作出版了具有深远影响的《通过公共政策促进健康》,其对《宪章》的问世具有重大意义[12]。在呼吁关注新的公共卫生之际,《宪章》认为提高健康水平需要充分支持、协调和促进卫生服务的重新定位,需要社会落实和个人技能相向而行,同时发力。为支持并强化这些健康促进战略,《宪章》主张制定健康的公共政策,即对各级政府采取的积极或者消极的卫生政策进行精准通盘的考虑[13]。《健康促进词汇》[14]将"健康的公共政策"描述为"对涉及健康和卫生公平的各领域政策通盘考虑,精准确定其健康影响。其主要目的是营造有利于人们健康生活的卫生环境。这样的政策让公众有更多的或更容易的健康选择,使社会环境和自然环境不断改善。"

Fafard 坚持这样的观点:"从国际和国内两个层面寻找在广泛的健康决定因素方面做出真正改变的政策和规划干预措施"是"令人费解的,因为这引出了一个能够包含世界上大多数政府正在作为(甚至是无力作为)的概念。"[15]Marmor 和 Boyum[16]甚至更为简洁地这样阐述:"认为确定某种不利于健康的因素——比

如贫穷——本身就能调动起来经济行动的想法是非常幼稚的。"

也许《宪章》和 Milio 关于政府全部门政策的健康影响潜力认定反映了一种理想主义时代精神,在这种精神的鼓舞下,人们坚定地相信基于理性和实证基础上的社会政策的作为与能量。但《宪章》留下的不朽遗产同样也显示了具有远见的观点拥有较大的影响力[17]。目前还几乎没有经验证据能够证明在缺少地方政府积极响应的情况下推行健康的公共政策的成功与失败[18]。大多数健康的公共政策的学术专著仍停留在抽象和修辞层面[19],没有政策研究基础和政治学基础[20]。

由于认识到健康决定因素不在卫生部门管理范围之内,已多次呼吁跨部门行动,正式开始于采纳《阿拉木图宣言》中的"初级卫生保健"观点,但在采纳《宪章》中的"健康促进"观点之后,这一呼声渐渐衰减。当另一种更为综合(平衡)的"初级卫生保健"观点认为该概念应框定于某些特定的疾病管理计划,这种呼声渐致萧条。

几十年来,世界卫生组织大力倡导并不断强调跨部门健康促进,如今真的需要落实起来以改善民众卫生福祉。一份 1986 年的报告[21]阐述了其他部门如何促进卫生事业发展。这份报告由世界卫生组织、联合国发展与国际经济合作总干事办公室、联合国环境规划署、联合国人类住区规划署和无家可归者收容安置国际年、联合国粮食及农业组织和联合国教科文组织联合发布。目前似乎仍然没有明显的进展,因为 2013 年第八届全球健康促进大会上的声明包括一系列类似的伙伴组织,比如经济合作与发展组织、联合国开发计划署、国际移民组织等,这些组织同样提出了相似的推荐和建议。引用 1986 年报告原文:"……应通过跨部门行动,为促进卫生事业发展调动一切潜在资源而付出努力。但现在还不能说,一个全面的跨部门方法能够使卫生部门同其他部门有效整合,从而塑造和影响健康相关方面朝着积极结果方向发展。"

自从这第一份试图在卫生领域融入其他部门协调配合的文件问世以来的 30年里,针对这一问题的言论也产生了一些实质性的发展。从不同的角度和领域,关于成立联合政府、整合型政府或综合治理的呼声持续不断。一些关于将分散的观点、管理办法、公共政策和产业规划集中整合[22]的综合性观点也开始出现。

三、把健康融入所有政策——仅仅停留在语言和修辞层面?

虽然 Milio 已经指出,社会生活的各方各面、公共政策和公民社会都会影响个人与群体的健康,但是以下领域对其的影响更为突出和持续:

- 教育；
- 住房和城市规划；
- 交通运输；
- 社会福利保障系统；
- 能源和可持续发展[23]。

世界各国各级政府都已试行综合卫生政策[24]。正是其中一些政策激发了《宪章》的发布，比如挪威的"农场-食品-营养"政策、中国的"赤脚医生"项目和美国的妇女健康倡议。两个来自地球两端的倡议开启了现在被称为"把健康融入所有政策"（Health in All Policies，HiAP）的发展进程。在担任欧盟轮值主席国期间，芬兰以其长期运营的北卡项目（名为"地平线健康计划"）的有效经验为基础，促请其他欧盟成员国加入：

"……一个平衡的、互补的政策相关的旨在提高公众健康福祉的战略。HiAP的核心在于研究一些主要受制于卫生领域以外政策的健康决定因素，通过调整这些因素，进而提高健康水平。"

几乎同时，南澳大利亚州政府在其思想家 Ilona Kickbusch 教授的指引下，出台了一系列政策和项目，用以投资其辖区的卫生事业：

"HiAP 旨在通过提高政府各部门政策的积极影响来改善民众健康福祉，同时也促进其他部门实现核心目标。"

这两项发展为第八届全球健康促进大会注入了强劲动力。大会通过了 HiAP 的宣言和框架：

"HiAP 是公共政策选择的一种方法，用以系统性权衡跨部门决策的健康影响，寻求协同，并避免给健康带来负面影响，从而促进公众健康并提高卫生公平。HiAP 可提升政策制定者在制定各层次政策时的卫生责任意识。它强调关注各公共政策对卫生系统、健康决定因素和居民身体健康所带来的影响。"

在不同的国家和行政辖区内，HiAP 各有侧重，但都有一个一贯的核心价值概念，那就是强调各公共政策制定部门的协调配合。至于不同国家和行政辖区内 HiAP 的不同点，主要包括卫生公平、协同效应实现方式、责任生成或责任驱使、创新应发挥的作用、政策综合的方式以及政策本身。比如[25]：

"HiAP 是一项协同性举措，通过在跨部门、各层级政策制定过程中清晰表达并综合考虑，进而提升全民健康福祉。"——美国国家和地区卫生官员协会（ASTHO）。

"HiAP 是一项通过在跨部门、跨领域政策制定过程中将卫生工作综合考虑进而提升全民健康福祉的协同性举措。"——加利福尼亚州 HiAP 督办处。

"HiAP 是在政策实施中包含、整合并协同考虑健康影响,尤其是在其他可能塑造或影响健康的社会决定因素的政策制定……HiAP 是领导人和政策制定者在制定、落实和评估各项政策时将健康、居民健康和社会公平综合考虑的政策实践。"——欧洲卫生系统和政策观察站。

"HiAP 具有其创新指向,在其推行进程中有关系统和工作方法自然产生变化,新的适应政策应运而生并得到落实。"——美国州与地区卫生官员协会(NACCHO)。

2014 年世界卫生大会决议 67.12("促进社会和经济发展:采取跨部门可持续行动促进健康和卫生公平")采纳了 HiAP 的建议。因而,全球范围内开启了磋商并审议这项政策进而保障其稳定推进和优先实施的热潮。HiAP 达到一个全球本土化发展高潮。

如上所述,HiAP 在经过几十年的发展后坚定地植根下来。期间从对医疗卫生发展、健康促进的思考到对健康和疾病的生成原因的复杂性探究,甚至对人类发展可持续性和顺应能力的前瞻性探索,再到地方、国家和全球层面对卫生公平的坚定支持,坚信不同种族、不同性别、不同发展阶段都应享有卫生公平。在联合国和世界卫生组织决议在全球和区域层面给予一致认定后,围绕这些问题的讨论开始向权利基础性和价值趋向性发展。

显然,正如《宪章》所认定的,HiAP 需要包括健康的基础性先决条件(和平、住所、教育、食物、收入、稳定的生态系统、可持续的资源、社会公正和公平),从而推进医疗卫生进入一个互联互通的发展时代。

各大领域的深入研究已然拉开帷幕,具有通过经济上可行且有利的方式影响公众健康的巨大潜力。我们需要留意的是,对健康的社会决定因素进行的跨部门经济评估往往不能处理现有的社会梯度所带来的分配公平问题;关于卫生挑战的经济论证似乎存在于关键政策框架,抑或定位于平衡公共政策的成功介入。

公众卫生面临的问题是如何带动其他部门促进健康和发展的双赢。一份世界卫生组织的报告[26]提出,在跨部门利益层面,有三种类型的介入(图3)。图3所示的韦恩图表明,需要对 HiAP 是什么、可以是什么、应该是什么形成一种更加定制化和差异化的视图。一些 HiAP 由卫生部门主导并拥有(类型 1);一些也许由卫生部门发起,但由卫生部门同其他部门共同拥有(类型 2);还有一些由其他部门拥有,但卫生部门或许也有投入(类型 3)。

在各种情况下,都有必要对部门思维的动力和阻力拥有一个清晰的认识。这有助于上述类型"建设性介入"的推动者模糊部门界限并超越孤立性思考。联合政府、整合型政府、协调型政府、平衡综合型政府和政府治理(与跨部门和 HiAP

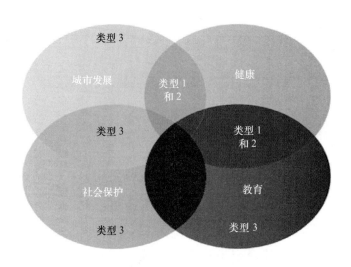

图3 部门间介入类型[26]

相呼应)等概念,自 20 世纪 70 年代就已从行政和政治科学里面衍生出来,而且自 20 世纪 80 年代以来就被多次尝试付诸实践和落实(从政府治理和行政管理角度)。发展如此全面的、连贯的方法(Peters[27] 称之为行政管理的"圣杯")的关键观念在于治理思想("通过一个由多维度互联互通建立起来的控制系统驾驭并协调一系列复杂的组织机构"[28])。良好的政府治理工具包括管控、协调、责任和权力[24]。但最重要的是,综合治理与政治有关[29]。政治系统(选民、议会、部长和官员,以及政治任命)似乎不能高效、优先地完成整合——要么因为整合过于复杂和排他,要么因为整合将会给其政治经济一体化发展带来挑战。

部门政策整合的障碍至少包括现有部门碎片化、责任缺失、部门利益固化、人际关系以及领导力。一些地方法律对整合有强制性要求——通常立法手段并不一定便利于物质执行条件——有时被称作实质性政策发展(非象征性政策),也就是说,将资源权责清晰地分配给制定目标的政策。

在向平衡综合型政府迈进的过程中,Peters[27] 指出了四条途径:① 通过所有利益攸关方参与的系统;② 通过认可和网络制度化;③ 通过成立部门行动价值导向协调机构;④ 通过扩展知识社群,使所有利益攸关方共同创造并利用知识。这些相当抽象的方法也许并不一定能够成功,尤其在一些综合卫生政策被认为是"动态目标"或"复杂的适应系统"的领域[30]:"一群可自由行动的个体往往会导致出人意料的局面,由于他们的行动彼此关联,因此其中一人的行动变化将会改变其他人行动的内容。"

关于通过公共部门整合促进卫生事业发展的文字表述一向不够明确。像"跨部门治理"[31]、"跨部门行动"[32]、"多部门行动"[33]、卫生公共政策和 HiAP 这类词汇都在混用着。

事实上，HiAP 作为一个概念已经在世界卫生组织和第八届全球健康促进大会上以结果文件及其必需背景文件的形式被标准化了[34]，世界卫生大会有关的跟进解决方案没有对 HiAP 进行热议，而是将其形容为"促进跨部门卫生行动和卫生公平的框架"[35]——这个概念框定就可以显示出卫生发展事业的综合举措是一个多么富有政治挑战性的领域。

然而，我们需要对（跨部门的、整合的等）治理、政策和落实进行概念区分，可以根据欧洲健康城市的有关证据进行[36]。表 1 所示为类型概述。跨部门治理是"个人和组织、公共部门和私营部门管理其共同事务方式的总和。这是一个持续的过程，通过这一进程，相互冲突的或者不同的利益会通过采取合作性方式得到妥善安置。这包括正式机构或制度授权的强制执行，也包括人们和机构之间或者达成一致或者感知到符合最大利益而达成的非正式协议。"（卫生）治理是一个无形的基于"我们是怎么做的"的价值和信念组合。就此我们需要一个决定性的定义，但目前还没有得到。在社会各个系统和个人行为之间经常上演的、现已确认的治理有三种类型[37]。根据 Leeuw、Clavier 和 Breton 的理论[38]，跨部门政策是"政府就通过相关因素分配资源和能力，进而在一定时间框架内解决意向已确认的卫生问题而表达的意向。"这往往通过管理、分配和重新分配三种形式体现。在对跨部门落实进行概念厘定时，将"落实"与政策工具在语言上联系起来似乎很有用处。政策工具"要么影响政策落实的内容，要么影响其过程。也就是说，政策工具或者调整商品和服务分配给公众的方式，或者调整这种分配落实的方法。"[39]但是政策工具在从困难厘定到结果评估的政策设计中发挥一定作用。跨部门政策工具箱包括（积极或消极）处置、创造便利设施和沟通性行动（也许不够严谨）。

表 1　（跨部门）治理、政策和落实（政策工具）的类型

治理	政策	落实
基本的	管理	处置
指导性的	分配	设施
操作性的	重新分配	沟通

或许总结得有些草率，"治理"是为游戏设定总规则，"政策"是解决问题的实质性决定，而"落实"是实现改变的工具。

在试图厘清这些关键概念时，我们不可否认，关于综合治理、政策和落实的实证研究是非常具有挑战性的。1988 年，在世界卫生组织欧洲地区 46 个国家相互交界地区，有学者第一次尝试就卫生综合治理做出系统性综述[40]。2015 年，一项就 99 个欧洲城市进行跟进描述的清单正式出版[41]。此类研究工作面临的挑战愈发清晰：工作规则的设定、各级政府之间的相互关联方式都各有不同，这给系统性研究带来了挑战，但我们总有更新颖的方法论，包括现实主义综合论[42]。

四、落实 HiAP 的举措

所以我们并不奇怪，现有的整合卫生治理、政策和落实的做法本质上常常是粗略的（基于一些遴选的特定案例的研究）、抽象的（基于理论和/或修辞）和任务性的（基于上级指示）。

在众多落实举措中，培训工作手册和能力建设工具这两个例子是相关的。世界卫生组织发布了 HiAP 的工作手册。手册中写道：

"考虑到政府对卫生工作应负的责任和当前卫生领域面临的许多复杂挑战，为落实 HiAP，政府部门需要做好但不局限于以下关键工作：

（1）委任研究；

（2）动员政府内外的利益相关方；

（3）制定并落实跨部门政策；

（4）评估其作用。"

手册采纳了"跨部门治理"观点持有者的建议，认为 HiAP 需要以下有关单位的支持：

（1）内阁委员会和秘书处；

（2）议会各委员会；

（3）跨部门委员会和有关单位；

（4）各部位合署办公机构；

（5）联合预算；

（6）跨部门政策制定支持；

（7）非政府利益相关方的参与。

为进一步推动上述工作机制的创建和持久运作，手册采纳了由 Leppo 等[43]提出的关于 HiAP 的几类观点：

（1）健康观点——健康具有其内生价值，政府部门能够而且应该支持其他公共事业管理部门参与并推动卫生事业发展。

（2）健康作用于其他部门观点——健康和卫生公平的改善可以助力其他部门在公共事业管理方面获得更多的政府授权。

（3）健康-社会目标观点——健康和卫生公平的发展可以增进社会各领域的获得感。

（4）经济观点——如前所述,健康有利于财富积累,促进经济社会发展。

一些证据表明,健康观点并不利于 HiAP 的推进。据调查,苏格兰受访者建议避免强调"健康"一词,当以构建环境可持续城市为出发点时,建设健康城市的目标自然在各部门的协同配合下实现了。

我们对推进 HiAP 进程的不同阶段进行了划分,从倡议、协调到程序化运作。各个阶段不同学术观点和实证经验相互重叠。HiAP 本身将领导力置于非常重要的位置,不仅是各部委、各机构首长的领导力,更是所有实践参与者和社区群众的领导力[44]。如前所述,关于综合卫生治理、卫生政策和卫生落实有很多见解深刻的分析和稳健有效的推行举措,尤其在世界卫生组织、南澳大利亚和芬兰。前文中概述了多维治理框架,并认为不同部门和"规则"能够而且应该适用于不同的理解层次,从而将不同的视角聚集在一起。我们也发现了一些能够证实上述观点的案例材料[45],使不同卫生政策达到相互理解可能的一个关键因素在于充分认可调研、政策和实践[46]之间的联系机制。最终,通过社群配合落实以及在"治理-政策-落实"范围内涌现的政治领导,HiAP 得到了持续性发展。为此,所有不同层次的有关机构都要将 HiAP 列入部门规定,并且依规执行。"自上而下"需要同"自下而上"相向而行,态性复杂需要专注分析。落实的圣杯已然触手可及,我们需要做的就是坚定不移地向前推进。

参 考 文 献

[1] MARMOT M. Social determinants of health inequalities. The Lancet, 2005,365(9464):1099-1104.

[2] BLUM H L. Planning for health: development and application of social change theory. Human Sciences Press.1974.

[3] LAFRAMBOISE H L. Health policy: breaking the problem down into more manageable segments. Canadian Medical Association Journal, 1973,108(3):388.

[4] EVANS R G, BARER M L, MARMOR T R. Why are some people healthy and others not? The determinants of the health of populations. Transaction Publishers. 1994.

[5] ERIKSSON M, LINDSTRÖM B. Antonovsky's sense of coherence scale and the relation with health: a systematic review. Journal of Epidemiology & Community Health, 2006,60(5):376-381.

[6] DAHLGREN G, WHITEHEAD M. Policies and strategies to promote equity in health. World Health Organization, Regional Office for Europe. 1992.

[7] GRAHAM H. Social determinants and their unequal distribution: clarifying policy understandings. The Milbank Quarterly, 2004,82(1):101-124.

[8] Canadian Council on Social Determinants of Health. A review of frameworks on the determinants of

health. 2015.

[9] MILIO N. Promoting health through public policy. Philadelphia：FA Davis Co.1981.

[10] HANCOCK T. Beyond health care：from public health policy to healthy public policy. Canadian Public Health Association, Ottawa. 1985.

[11] DE LEEUW E, CLAVIER C. Healthy public in all policies. Health Promotion International,2011,26(suppl 2)：ii237-244.

[12] World Health Organization, Health Canada, Canadian Public Health Association. The Ottawa charter for health promotion：the move towards a new public health. 1986.

[13] World Health Organization. Adelaide recommendations for healthy public policy. 1988.

[14] NUTBEAM D. Health promotion glossary. Health Promotion International,1998,13：349-364.

[15] FAFARD P. Evidence and healthy public policy：insights from health and political sciences. Canadian Policy Research Networks May. 2008.

[16] MARMOR T R, BOYUM D. Medical care and public policy：the benefits and burdens of asking fundamental questions. Health Policy (Amsterdam, Netherlands),1999,49：27-43.

[17] HANCOCK T. Health promotion in Canada：25 years of unfulfilled promise. Health Promotion International, 2011, 26(suppl 2)：ii263-267.

[18] DE LEEUW E, GREEN G, SPANSWICK L, et al. Policymaking in European healthy cities. Health Promotion International,2015,30：i18-31.

[19] BOWMAN S, UNWIN N, CRITCHLEY J, et al. Use of evidence to support healthy public policy: a policy effectiveness-feasibility loop. Bulletin of the World Health Organization,2012,90：847-853.

[20] BRETON E, DE LEEUW E. Theories of the policy process in health promotion research：a review. Health Promotion International,2011,26：82-90.

[21] World Health Organization. Intersectoral action for health：the role of intersectoral cooperation in national strategies for health for all.1986.

[22] CHRISTENSEN T, LÆGREID P. The whole-of-government approach to public sector reform. Public Administration Review,2007,67：1059-1066.

[23] DE LEEUW E. Engagement of sectors other than health in integrated health governance, policy, and action. Annual Review of Public Health, 2017,38：329-349.

[24] DE LEEUW E. From urban projects to healthy city policies//DE LEEUW E, SIMOS J. Healthy Cities—The Theory, Policy, and Practice of Value-based Urban Planning. Springer. 2017：407-437.

[25] RUDOLPH L, CAPLAN J, BEN-MOSHE K, et al. Health in all policies：a guide for state and local governments. American Public Health Association and Public Health Institute. 2013.

[26] WHO. The economics of the social determinants of health and health inequalities：a resource book. 2013.

[27] PETERS B G. Managing horizontal government：the politics of co-ordination. Public Administration,1998, 76：295-311.

[28] FLINDERS M. Governance in Whitehall. Public Administration,2002, 80：51-75.

[29] DE LEEUW E, PETERS D. Nine questions to guide development and implementation of Health in All Policies. Health Promotion International,2015,30：987-997.

［30］ PLSEK P E, GREENHALGH T. Complexity science: the challenge of complexity in health care. BMJ, 2001,323: 625-628.

［31］ MCQUEEN D, WISMAR M, LIN V, et al. Intersectoral governance for health in all policies: structures, actions and experiences. Copenhagen: World Health Organization Regional Office for Europe. 2012.

［32］ MARMOT M, ALLEN J J. Social determinants of health equity. American Journal of Public Health,2014, 104(suppl 4):517-519.

［33］ World Health Organization. Global action plan for the prevention and control of noncommunicable diseases 2013-2020. 2013.

［34］ PUSKA P, STÅHL T. Health in all policies—the finnish initiative: background, principles, and current issues. Annual review of public health,2010,31: 315-328.

［35］ World Health Assembly. Resolution WHA67.12 Contributing to social and economic development: sustainable action across sectors to improve health and health equity. 2014.

［36］ DE LEEUW E. Intersectoral action, policy and governance in European Healthy Cities. Public Health Panorama,2015, 1(2):175-182.

［37］ HILL M, HUPE P. Analysing policy processes as multiple governance: accountability in social policy. Policy Politics,2006,34:557-573.

［38］ DE LEEUW E, CLAVIER C, BRETON E. Health policy—why research it and how: health political science. Health Research Policy and Systems,2014,12(1):55.

［39］ HOWLETT M. Managing the "hollow state": procedural policy instruments and modern governance. Canadian Public Administration. 2000: 412-431.

［40］ GREEN G. Health and governance in European cities: a compendium of trends and responsibilities for public health in 46 member states of the WHO European Region. European Hospital Management Journal. 1988.

［41］ DE LEEUW E, PALMER N, SPANSWICK L. City fact sheets: WHO European Healthy Cities Network. Copenhagen: World Health Organization Regional Office for Europe. 2015.

［42］ DE LEEUW E, GREEN G, DYAKOVA M, et al. European healthy cities evaluation: conceptual framework and methodology. Health Promotion International, 2015,30(suppl 1):i8-17.

［43］ LEPPO K, OLLILA E, PENA S, et al. Health in all policies:seizing opportunities, implementing policies. Helsinki: Ministry of Social Affairs and Health. 2013.

［44］ GREER S L, LILLYIS D F. Beyond leadership: political strategies for coordination in health policies. Health Policy,2014,116(1):12-17.

［45］ SHANKARDASS K, SOLAR O, MURPHY K, et al. A scoping review of intersectoral action for health equity involving governments. International Journal of Public Health,2012,57: 25-33.

［46］ DE LEEUW E. From research to policy and practice in public health//LIAMPUTTONG P. Public Health: Local and Global Perspectives. Cambridge University Press,2016:213-234.

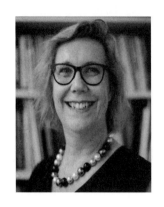

Eyelyne de Leeuw CHETRE 主任、《国际健康促进》杂志主编，世界卫生组织马斯特里赫特大学健康城市研究协作中心前任主任，迪肯大学和拉特巴大学名誉教授，蒙特利尔大学和马斯特里赫特大学客座教授，世界卫生组织欧洲健康城市研究中心主任。

2030 更健康:《全球公共卫生宪章》 与可持续发展目标

Michael Moore

世界公共卫生联盟

世界公共卫生联盟(WFPHA)与世界卫生组织(WHO)以及包括许多国际非政府组织在内的利益攸关方合作制定了《全球公共卫生宪章》(以下简称《宪章》)[1]。《宪章》旨在摆脱以疾病为中心的政策,并通过"预防、保护和健康促进"为改善健康提供指导。为此,《宪章》确定了四大推动力——能力建设、良好的治理、信息和宣传。

《宪章》的制定旨在与可持续发展目标(SDGs)相契合[2]。所有联合国成员国都承诺落实可持续发展目标。因此,将《宪章》作为协助落实可持续发展目标的途径并明确其重要性十分关键。

一、保　　护

可持续发展目标 13:保护人类健康不受气候风险影响,通过低碳发展促进健康

时任世界卫生组织总干事的陈冯富珍博士向世界公共卫生联盟提出制定《宪章》时,她对于改善健康的目标所面临的广泛挑战表示很担忧。改善全球健康所面临的巨大挑战不仅需要适时的行动,更需要一个合适的行动框架。总干事在WHO 执行委员会第 130 届会议的闭幕发言中说道:"公共卫生以及我们生活的整个世界所面临的挑战已经变得太多且太复杂了,现行措施已无法应对。"[3]

健康保护是《宪章》的三大重点内容之一。

(1) 全球健康是国家间协调的关键因素。健康无国界。考虑到这一点,《国际卫生条例》是"一项对全球 196 个国家包括 WHO 所有成员国具有约束力的国际法律文书"[4]。该条例提出了人口保护的一个重要方面,即只有通过适当的协调才能实现。

63

（2）传染病控制也是一个全球性问题，中国在"禽流感"和"猪流感"暴发中的经验、影响和领导作用一直是各国应对传染病与开展国际预防的关键元素[5]。

（3）应急防范与传染病预防并行不悖。从西非埃博拉疫情、海啸、地震和其他突发事件中汲取的经验教训提醒我们如果缺乏应对突发事件的能力将会发生什么。

（4）地球健康是保护的关键元素。这一概念包括：环境健康、气候变化和可持续性。"地球健康是指人类文明及其所赖以生存的自然系统的健康。"[6]

（5）气候行动是地球健康的关键因素之一。气候变化是国际社会健康面临的最大挑战之一。

特朗普总统宣布退出《巴黎协定》，表示他"代表匹兹堡市民，而非巴黎市民"，似乎是美国这个世界上最大的污染者之一正在制造一场全球性灾难[7]。然而，要记住的是，美国国内进行了一场声势浩大的运动，州长们和市长们在2017年6月结成了美国气候联盟，涉及10个州的274个城市[8]。

太平洋地区也发生了类似的事情。澳大利亚面临着进一步采矿的威胁，而特恩布尔政府却支持印度企业阿达尼公司在卡米高开发新的煤矿，该煤矿将是世界上最大的煤矿之一[9]。这对气候行动的威胁是切实而紧迫的。

与此同时，太平洋小国将首当其冲受到影响。在南太平洋大学等联合主办的联合国政府间气候变化专门委员会（IPCC）会议上，人们对《联合国气候变化框架公约》（UNFCCC）甚至整个世界表示担忧，不知道问题到底有多么严峻，应采取何种紧急行动来挽救我们的岛屿、我们的土地、我们的人民、文化，以及最终——我们的国家"[10]。

二、预防

可持续发展目标12：负责任的消费和生产

《宪章》认为，预防应更加广泛地包括：① 一级预防——疫苗接种；② 二级预防——筛查；③ 三级预防——以证据为基础且以社区为基础的、综合性的、以人为本的优质医疗和康复服务；④ 医疗管理和计划。

在根据可持续发展目标进行审查时，可依据可持续发展目标12"负责任的消费和生产"来考虑《宪章》的预防重点。

（1）抗微生物药物耐药性（AMR）已成为一个国际挑战，部分原因是不负责任的消费。在澳大利亚，有人预测，到2050年，抗微生物药物耐药性将超过癌症成为致死的主要原因[11]。作者指出，"由于细菌可跨境传播，抗微生物药物耐药性将迅速传播且不易被发现，因此这一问题应得到全球的普遍关注"。

（2）负责任消费的其他挑战包括烟草、垃圾食品和酒精。① 菲利普·莫里斯烟草公司想让我们相信，它是一只已经改变了豹纹的豹子，致力于构建"无烟世界"[12]。该公司一边向发展中国家推销致命产品（按指示使用，导致三分之二的人比不吸烟者早 10 年死亡[13]），一边表明未经证实的电子香烟和 IQOS 电子烟将有助于形成"无烟世界"。伪善得令人恐惧！烟草能致命。但通过其他设备将超细颗粒吸入肺部的危害证据尚未明晰。② 肥胖仍然是一个全球性挑战，国际大企业所推动的消费风险很高，这意味着下一代人将首次成为近几个世纪里比当代人生活得更不健康且寿命更短的一代人。③ 有害使用酒类饮品也成为一大挑战，不健康的消费为国际公司带来了丰厚的利润。有害使用酒类饮品会导致从肝脏和心血管病到癌症的一系列疾病。同时，这也是暴力事件的一个重要催化剂。

（3）如果不希望健康（或不健康）议程由重利益、轻健康的国际公司制定的话，就需要各国政府进行良好治理。负责任的消费方面，良好的政府治理意味着：

① 通过恰当的市场营销、准确信息和有效标签等干预措施促进健康消费[14]。

② 政府要在限制不健康产品的营销中发挥重要作用。售酒公司赞助赛车运动就是一个例子。驾驶与酒精之间的有害关系众所周知，应严厉禁止国内和国际上的此类营销。

③ 抵制关于"保姆式国家"的争论对于公共卫生也至关重要[15]。政府干预要比让大型国际公司制定健康议程好得多。

三、健康促进

可持续发展目标 1：优先考虑穷人的健康需求

可持续发展目标 10：减少不平等

《宪章》中关于健康促进的内容源于《健康促进渥太华宪章》，并融入了最新进展。其包括以下问题：不平等、环境决定因素、社会和经济决定因素、弹性、行为和健康素养、生命周期，以及健康的环境。

（1）在 WHO"可持续发展时代的健康"中，可持续发展目标 1 提到"优先考虑穷人的健康需求"，可持续发展目标 10 提到"减少不平等"。这些是落实《宪章》的关键因素。不幸的是，世界正朝着相反的方向前行，富人越来越富，而穷人越来越穷。对于那些有意改善全人类健康状况的人来说，国际、国家和地方层面的不断扩大的差距是一个关键挑战。乐施会 2017 年 1 月发布的报告和其他关于财富不平等的报告都提出了严峻的警告[16]。在国际上，即使是一个不可思议的发现也能清晰地反映出我们所面临的挑战。"8 位亿万富豪的财富就相当于最贫困的36 亿人的财富总和"。在澳大利亚，也有一个类似的例子："1% 的澳大利亚人拥有着相当于 70% 底层人民的财富"。全球有"十分之一的人每天仅靠不足 2 美元来维持生计"。

（2）国际乐施会清楚地表明，"为了让本就富有的股东获得更大的回报，大型企业正在避税、压低工人工资和生产者价格，并减少对企业的投资"。

四、良好的治理

可持续发展目标 3：良好健康与福祉

《宪章》指出，良好的治理是产生公平的健康成果的关键因素。其中包括：公共卫生立法、健康和跨部门政策、策略、融资、组织、保证、透明度、问责和审计。在审查"可持续发展目标时代的卫生"时，要重点关注可持续发展目标 3"良好健康与福祉"。这一部分可分为挑战和希望。

（一）挑战

（1）挑战包括孕产妇死亡率。虽然过去 50 年间全球孕产妇死亡率已有极大改善，但分布不均，仍有大量社区中的分娩母亲的健康结果极差。

（2）艾滋病、肺结核（包括抗生素耐药性）、疟疾以及许多其他疾病仍然是国际社会面临的严峻挑战。然而，这些疾病的主要挑战仍是贫穷的根本问题。公共卫生的基础就是了解健康的社会决定因素。

（3）非传染性疾病日益严重。肥胖不再只与发达经济体有关。现在，中低收入国家的医疗保健成本、发病率和死亡率都在大幅上升。这一挑战被视为"威胁世界各地"的"肥胖海啸"[17]。

（4）与交通事故有关的发病率和死亡率在发达国家中正在下降，但在中低收入国家中却正在上升。应对此类健康负担的措施已经明确，亟须落实。

（二）希望

（1）《烟草控制框架公约》为应对与吸烟有关的疾病和死亡提供了明确的方向。澳大利亚是世界上烟草使用量最低的国家之一。2016 年，只有 2% 的青少年是非吸烟者，而在澳大利亚各年龄段人群中，只有 12% 是每日吸烟者[18]。一些国家已经采取了多方面措施减少吸烟，这些措施可在其他吸烟率高的国家进行推广。

（2）疫苗接种仍是解决传染病最有效的方法之一。天花已通过免疫接种被彻底消除，世界正站在消灭小儿麻痹症的边缘。扶轮国际、WHO、全球疫苗免疫联盟、盖茨基金会正在与政府、非政府组织和个人共同努力，并且逐步取得进展。

2017年12月数据显示，当年野生脊髓灰质炎病毒感染病例数为17例，较上一年减少一半[19]。

（3）国际条约对健康有重大影响。虽然仍有诸多挑战，但世界贸易组织在2001年就明确了健康问题的重要性。《多哈宣言》试图解决"政府运用公共卫生原则和《与贸易有关的知识产权协定》（TRIPS）的条款的需求"[20]。其中一个关键要素就是要找到合适的方法，确保更公平地获得基本药物和保健品。

五、准确的信息

可持续发展目标4：支持开展高质量的全民教育，以改善健康和公平

《宪章》深入阐明了准确信息的重要性和影响力。在公共卫生方面，这意味着确保参与监管、监督和评估，监测健康决定因素，研究与证据，风险与创新，传播与吸收。

（1）"可持续发展时代的健康"中的例子是可持续发展目标4，旨在支持"开展高质量的全民教育，以改善健康和公平"。《宪章》表明，决策要基于最佳证据。

（2）不仅证据至关重要，解释健康政策并使其在社会各阶层之间传播也至关重要。开展公开的公共卫生辩论时，基于证据，有助于消除关于疫苗接种、赌博等不健康活动，以及烟酒、垃圾食品等不健康消费的误区。

（3）这种辩论为确定公共卫生政策失败的经济成本提供了机会，其不仅影响人民健康，也影响国家的生产力和国内生产总值。

（4）监督和评估也是衡量成功的关键因素。用WHO前总干事陈冯富珍博士的话说："正如我常说的那样，所测即所得。"[3]

（5）但是，仅有监督是不够的。利用传统媒体和社交媒体传播健康信息已成为公共卫生的一个关键因素。那些宣传不健康的活动和商品的公司目前正在大量使用这种方法，为了实现2030年更健康的未来，我们需要予以反击。

六、能　力　建　设

可持续发展目标6：清洁用水和卫生设施

公共卫生能力建设是改善全球健康状况的关键因素。这个概念需要政府、非政府组织、大学和其他教育机构以及所有公共卫生专业人员承担责任。《宪章》明确了能力建设的关键领域：公共卫生人力开发、卫生工作者和更广泛的劳动力；劳动力规划（数量、资源、基础设施）；标准、课程、认证；能力、教学和培训。

（1）能力建设方面要用到的例子是"可持续发展时代的健康"中的目标6，即"清洁用水和卫生设施"。这个目标是最基本的。这是公共卫生和流行病学学生面临的问题，也是他们课程学习的第一部分。

（2）John Snow 和牧师 Henry Whitehead 在英国进行的第一个流行病学研究的故事成了许多流行病学文献的第一章[21]。然而，这些文章往往止步于发现霍乱通过宽街的水泵进行传播。不常提及的故事是，尽管英国政府利用他们的证据在伦敦和全国各地引入下水道，但行动的催化剂实际上是 1858 年伦敦的"大恶臭"。由于臭气熏天无法抵挡，威斯敏斯特议会无法解决。这种情况下，议员们利用证据，找到了采取行动的适当方式。由此可见，公共卫生具有政治性。

（3）WHO 与联合国儿童基金会于 2017 年发布的一份联合报告[22]表明，"90个国家中的基本卫生设施建设进展过于缓慢，这意味着到 2030 年，无法实现卫生设施的全覆盖"。此外，"全世界约有十分之三的人无法在家中获得安全、清洁的水，还有五分之三的人缺乏安全管理的卫生设施"。

（4）一个半世纪以来，我们已经知道了清洁用水和卫生设施对于健康的重要性，但能力却仍不足。因此，政治行动成为推进这一工作的重要手段。

七、高 效 宣 传

可持续发展目标 17：动员各合作伙伴监督和实现与健康相关的可持续发展目标

高效宣传已被世界公共卫生联盟确定为促进健康的关键因素。高效宣传的效果远好于"游说"。其中包括：领导力与道德、健康公平、社会动员与团结、公众教育、以人为本的方针、自愿社区参与、通信，以及可持续发展。

（1）动员各合作伙伴来监督和实现与健康相关的可持续发展目标是"可持续发展时代的健康"中引用的最后一个例子。

（2）世界公共卫生联盟在全世界拥有超过 120 个成员，并与广泛的利益攸关方进行合作，为国际社会创造更好的健康结果。这意味着全球有超过 100 万人对公共卫生有着浓厚的兴趣。世界公共卫生联盟的目标是"为所有人争取健康公平和健康长寿的生活"。该团体是"国际性的、非政府性的民间团体与多学科公共卫生联盟，致力于疾病预防和公众健康的促进和保护"。

（3）30 年前成立的中华预防医学会（CPMA）是世界公共卫生联盟的成员之一，在中国、西太平洋地区乃至国际上，对于改善健康结果都有极大影响力。中华预防医学会负责世界公共卫生联盟在西太平洋地区的工作，并与整个地区的公共卫生协会进行合作，促进互联、能力建设和宣传。

（4）中华预防医学会也是世界公共卫生联盟理事会的积极成员，通过有效的政策和明智的参与来实现更好的健康结果。

（5）世界公共卫生联盟与 WHO 已建立正式关系。《宪章》的发展便源自于这种关系。通过这种关系和其他许多关系，诸多机遇展现在世界公共卫生联盟及其成员协会面前。高效宣传的关键因素之一是管理伙伴关系，从而提升影响力[23]。

八、结论

中华预防医学会成立 30 年来，中国卫生事业取得了长足发展，但在确保公平的健康结果、增强预防和保护、加强健康促进等方面仍然任重道远。作为落实可持续发展目标的一种手段，公共卫生协会、各国政府和相关行业可以运用一系列重要的工具来实现更好的保护、预防和健康促进。《宪章》将这些工具确定为：良好的治理、能力建设、准确信息和宣传。

上述例子说明了《宪章》与可持续发展目标之间的关系。不过，这只是一部分例子。《宪章》有望助力落实更广泛的可持续发展目标。鉴于各国政府对落实可持续发展目标做出的承诺，《宪章》可成为用于协助落实工作的重要工具。

参 考 文 献

[1] LOMAZZI M A. Global charter for the public's health—the public health system：role，functions，competencies and education requirements. Eur J Public Health，2016，26（2）：210-212.

[2] UN. Sustainable Development Goals 2017. 2017.

[3] CHAN M. WHO Director General Addresses the Executive Board. 2012.

[4] WHO. International Health Regulations 2007. 2017.

[5] YANG W Z. Early warning for infectious disease outbreak theory and practice. London：Elsevier，2017.

[6] HORTON R，LO S. Planetary health：a new science for exceptional action. Lancet，2015，386（10007）：1921-1922.

[7] WATTS M. Cities spearhead climate action. Nature Climate Change，2017，7：537-538.

[8] MINDOCK C. Paris agreement：US states and mayors fight climate change after Donald Trump pulls US out of deal. 2017.

[9] HOLMES D. Australia's climate bomb：the senselessness of Adani's Carmichael coal mine. 2017.

[10] University of the South Pacific. USP co-hosts Fiji's inaugural Lead Authors Meeting for IPCC. 2017.

[11] KELLY R，DAVIES S C. Tackling antimicrobial resistance globally. Med J Aust，2017，207（9）：371-373.

[12] WHO. WHO statement on Philip Morris funded foundation for a smoke-free world. 2017.

[13] BANKS E，JOSHY G，WEBER M F，et al. Tobacco smoking and all-cause mortality in a large Australian cohort study：findings from a mature epidemic with current low smoking prevalence. BMC Medicine，2015，13（1）：38.

[14] TALATI Z，NORMAN R，PETTIGREW S，et al. The impact of interpretive and reductive front-of-pack labels on food choice and willingness to pay. International Journal of Behavioral Nutrition and Physical Activity，

2017,14(1):171.

[15] MOORE M, YEATMAN H DAVEY R. Which nanny—the state or industry? Wowsers, teetotallers and the fun police in public health advocacy. Public Health, 2015,129(8):1030-1037.

[16] Oxfam International. An economy for the 99 percent. 2017.

[17] WISE J. "Tsunami of obesity" threatens all regions of world, researchers find. BMJ,2011, 342:772.

[18] AIHW. Teenage smoking and drinking down, while drug use rises among older people. 2017.

[19] GPEI. Polio global eradication initiative. 2017.

[20] WHO. The Doha declaration on the TRIPS agreement and public health. 2017.

[21] HENNEKENS C H, BURING J E. Epidemiology in medicine. Little Brown and Company,1987.

[22] WHO/UNICEF. Progress on drinking water, sanitation and hygiene:2017 update and sustainable development goal. 2017.

[23] MOORE M, YEATMAN H, POLLARD C. Evaluating success in public health advocacy strategies. Vietnam Journal of Public Health,2013,1(1):66-75.

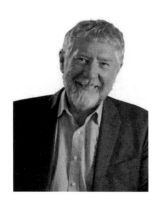

Michael Moore　澳大利亚公共卫生首席执行官，世界公共卫生联盟主席，前卫生和社区护理部长，澳大利亚首都地区立法大会独立成员(1989—2001年)，澳大利亚勋章获得者(勋爵)。悉尼科技大学客座教授，堪培拉大学兼职教授。

Part I

Overview

Overview

WANG Longde, YANG Weizhong, LIU Xia, TIAN Chuansheng, XIN Meizhe, XIA Jianguo, YANG Peng, CUI Zengwei

Chinese Preventive Medicine Association

1　Forum overview

From 18th to 19th November 2017, International Top-level Forum on Engineering Science and Technology Development Strategy—Healthy China was successfully held in Beijing, with the theme of "Health in All Policies". The forum welcomed more than 2000 experts, scholars, professionals, technicians and representatives from Chinese Academy of Engineering (CAE), China Association for Science and Technology (CAST), National Health and Family Planning Commission (NHFPC), medical institutions of all levels, scientific research institutions, institutions of higher learning, and health related associations and enterprises

The opening ceremony was hosted by YANG Weizhong, the Vice President and Secretary General of Chinese Preventive Medicine Association (CPMA). The opening ceremony was addressed by WANG Longde who is the President of the forum, Member of Deputy Director level of Education, Science, Culture and Health Committee of the 12th NPC, President of CPMA and Academician of Chinese Academy of Engineering, HAN Qide who is the Vice President of CPPCC and Honorary President of CAST represented by SONG Jun who is the Member of the Party Leadership Group and Director of Association and Academic Division and concurrently of Enterprise Office of CAST, WANG Guoqiang who is the Deputy Minister of NHFPC and Director General of State Administration of Traditional Chinese Medicine, LIU Xu who is the Vice President of CAE, Michael Moore who is the President of World Federation of Public Health Associations (WFPHA) and Fabio Scano who is the coordinator of World Health Organization(WHO)

China Office. They called on all the sectors of the society to adhere to the working principle of Prevention Playing the Main Role, closely connect with and provide services to the strategy of Healthy China, and thus make contributions to push the construction of Healthy China. Academician LI Lanjuan, Academician ZHANG Boli and officials from related departments attended the awarding ceremony for scientific and technological progress and other activities of CPMA during the opening ceremony.

The International Top-level Forum on Engineering Science and Technology Development Strategy—Healthy China invited 6 academicians of CAE including WANG Longde, LIU Xu, WEI Yu, CHEN Junshi, GAO Runlin and ZHONG Nanshan, as well as 3 internationally renowned experts including Evelyne de Leeuw, Timo Stahl and Michael Moore to make reports during the forum. Academician CHEN Junshi and Prof. CHEN Yude as well as Researcher WANG Yu and Prof. Evelyne de Leeuw hosted the morning and afternoon sessions respectively. With the focus of "Health in All Policies", the academicians had an in-depth description of the concepts and paths towards constructing a healthy China and shared Chinese wisdom and cases from the perspective of developing people with health concepts in mind, optimizing health related services and improving health related policies. Foreign experts introduced the progress in global health campaign and its successful experience, and clearly explained the indicators of the health sector in 2030 Sustainable Development Goals (SDGs). Academician WANG Longde made the summary at the closing ceremony.

The 5th Academic Annual Meeting of CPMA was also held at the same time; it invited more than 200 experts to make themed reports at 27 parallel sessions. More than 500 papers were discussed and nearly 50 elected as excellent during the annual meeting, covering prevention and cure of chronic diseases, health emergency, health evaluation and management, health promotion and education, vaccines and immune system, epidemiology, early life development and disease control, prevention and cure of adult diseases for children and other hot-spot and difficult issues in the health sector. Awards were presented during the meeting including the Science and Technology Award of CPMA in 2017, the 2015-2016 Excellent Journal Award and Excellent Journal Worker Award of CPMA in 2017, the best practice of chronic disease prevention and cure in China, the popular science book of the 1st Healthy China · Scientific China— Project for Promoting Excellent Popular Science Books of Chronic Disease Prevention and Control in China, and the 1st National Moms' Excellent Popular Science Videos.

Three solicitation drafts were issued during the meeting, including "History of Public Health and Preventive Medicine in China", "China in 2049: Science and Technology and Society Vision—Preventive Medicine and Quality of Life", "Health Report of Chinese People in 2016". Summary and Commendation Conference of FPFD (female pelvic floor dysfunction) Prevention and Cure in China was also held at the same time.

The forum is a grand gathering held after the successful convening of the 19th National Congress of CPC to implement the strategy of Healthy China. The meeting had drawn special attention from institutions and professionals in the health sector. HAN Qide, Vice President of CPPCC, specially sent a written speech to the meeting. More than 100 domestic and foreign institutions sent congratulatory messages to the successful convening of the meeting with 10 academicians sending inscription or dedication. It enjoyed a live coverage by more than 20 media including Xinhua News Agency, Health News, Science and Technology Daily, people.com.cn, gmw.com.cn, China.com.cn, cnr.cn and cctv.com; it was also live broadcasted by the official website and Wechat account of CPMA, gmw.cn and other platforms, plus 6 academicians and more than 10 renowned experts received live interview regarding hot-spot and popular science issues in the health sector, viewed by more than 1.1 million people.

2 Experts' speeches and discussions

WANG Longde, President of the forum and President of CPMA, first made the report named "Strategy as a Priority for the Healthy China Initiative". He pointed out that currently, China has achieved significantly in the reform of the health sector with continuous improvement of people's health conditions and physical quality. However, there is still a clear contradiction between the insufficient supply of services in health sector and the increasing demand. The coordination of development between the health sector and the economy and society need to be strengthened, and major and long-term issues need to be addressed from the perspective of national strategy. Therefore, China needs to be clear to implement Healthy China Strategy, improving health related policies for the public and providing all-round health services to the public from the very beginning to the end; the *Healthy China 2030 Planning Outline* also proposes the development strategies and targets in two phases, as well as a series of concrete indicators and requirements. Policy goes first in constructing a Healthy China. He also shared his practices of developing strategies and ideas in the aspect of the legislation regarding integrating health concepts into all the policies, health related technology and strategy and popularization of applicable technology.

Afterwards, LIU Xu, Vice President of CAE, analyzed the trend of food supply and consumption in China and its relationship with health in his report "Agriculture, Food Development and National Nutrition Health". He suggested that agricultural development and national nutrition and health can be improved from three aspects namely agricultural supply side, demand side and macro-control. From the agricultural supply side, it still needs to continuously increase total food supply and improve quality; from the demand side, efforts should be made to promote dietary guidelines, increase consumption and assistance of certain kinds of food and supervise and direct food consumption; from macro-control, governments of all levels should strengthen guidance and support of food and nutrition related work.

WEI Yu, the Former Vice Minister of Ministry of Education, made the report "Following the Law of Brain Development to Foster Healthy and Excellent Future Generations". In the report, she stressed that the period from pregnancy to 3 years old is an important phase for one's life development. In this period, there are good opportunities to promote life's development; however, it is also a sensitive period of time when infants in different dire situations suffer from negative impacts. Not only do malnutrition and harm of various kinds bring severe consequences, but also an education environment filled with negligence brings great harm to the children. Thus, their brains' development process are changed, which influence their life-long health conditions, increase the possibility of getting diseases and lower the cognitive competence. She therefore suggested that the country should forward the focus of poverty alleviation time to the first 1000 days of a person. Poverty alleviation efforts in medicine, education and other aspects should be integrated to support and improve the education environment of children in poor families, and carry out an integrated campaign to help children living under poverty line. It is also an effective measure to promote targeted poverty alleviation, realize fair education and sever intergenerational pass of poverty.

Academician CHEN Junshi from China National Center for Food Safety Risk Assessment made the report "Better Nutrition for a Healthy China". He pointed out that nutrition level is closely connected to health and disease of the Chinese people, and that nutriology is a necessity to implement the *Healthy China 2030 Planning Outline* and build a moderately prosperous society in all respects. He began from explaining the latest health related policies, the *Healthy China 2030 Planning Outline* and other documents, and then analyzed the background of issuing *National Nutrition Plan 2017–2030*. He then pointed out that the concepts of nutrition and health are in the best time of policy, and that the implementation of related plans will definitely make great contributions to build a moderately prosperous society in all respects and realize the dream of Healthy China.

Academician GAO Runlin from National Center for Cardiovascular Diseases made the report "Current Status and Prevention Strategy of Cardiovascular Diseases in China". He pointed out that cardiovascular diseases are the primary factor causing deaths of urban and rural residents and the death rate still has a rising trend. The increasing death rate is mainly caused by the aging population and prevalence of risks represented by high blood pressure, hypercholesteremia, diabetes, smoking, obesity, and so on. The key to preventing and curing such diseases is to prevent and control risk factors. The government should lead the effort, make prevention as the central task, standardize and guarantee the implementation of prevention and cure management, establish layered diagnosis and treatment system, promote the transfer from medical insurance to health insurance and give full play to "Internet +". He stressed that an early arrival of the turning point of the death rate in an effort to prevent and cure cardiovascular diseases will be greatly accelerated through integrating health concepts into all the policies, strengthening communication and coordination among different sectors and departments and performing comprehensive control of hypertension, hyperglycemia and hyperlipemia.

Academician ZHONG Nanshan, the Director of National Clinical Research Center for Respiratory Disease, made the report "Healthy China—Early Treatment Strategy for Respiratory Diseases". He began from explaining chronic respiratory diseases that account for 11% of the total deaths in China, and then pointed out that severe air pollution, smoking, and frequent major infectious respiratory diseases are the three major factors. He took the diagnosis and control of lung cancer and chronic obstructive pulmonary diseases as examples to illustrate that we should implement health related guidelines to realize early prevention and intervention of clinical diseases.

Prof. Evelyne de Leeuw, the Editor-in-Chief of *Health Promotion International*, made the report "Health in All Policies—Why and How". She specially emphasized that health is influenced by many factors, and that in the same sense, integrating health concepts into all the policies is also influenced by different social factors, including governance, policies, intervention, etc. Community is an important part through all the process.

Prof. Timo Stahl of Finland National Public Health Institute introduced the successful practice of Finland to Health in All Policies. In the report, Prof. Timo specially introduced the history, specific approaches and experience and lessons of integrating health concepts into all the policies proposed by Finland to EU. Their experience is that first there should be long-term investment and plan. Integrating health concepts into all the policies cannot be finished in a move and it requires expertise of public health and communication. All the people need to be involved. It should include not only physicians and but also other people. There should be data. Data concerning health and its determining factors should be integrated to analyze the relationship between health results, determining factors and policies. The awareness of public institutions, policymakers, media and civil servants need to be strengthened. Inter-department structural procedures and tools are also needed to realize a more systematic integration of health concepts into all the policies. These tools can help us realize and solve problems, make decisions and make arrangements among different departments. The Finnish practice proves that legislation support is very useful.

Dr. Michael Moore, the President of WFPHA, made the report "Better health by 2030: *The Global Charter* and the Sustainable Development Goals". He specially introduced *The Global Charter* jointly formulated by WFPHA, WHO and many other stakeholders including numerous international non-governmental organizations. As an approach to help realize UN SDGs, the Charter aims to get rid of disease centered policies, and provide guidance to improve health through "prevention, protection and health promotion". The four drivers are capacity building, good governance, information and advocacy. The report also resorted to some of the examples of UN SDGs, such as protecting health from climate risks, and promoting health through low-carbon development; responsible consumption and production; giving priority to consider health needs of the poor and reduce inequalities; good health and well-being; clean water and sanitation. These examples explain how to achieve greater health results for SDGs through utilizing the key factors of the Charter, taking a series of more concrete and practical measures and integrating health concepts into all the policies.

These experts come from different sectors and have very high academic attainments. With senior management experience in multiple important departments and organizations, they focused on the theme of Healthy China, and made the reports in the topics of health legislation, strengthening national nutrition level, focusing on children's early development and implementing early diagnosis and cure strategy of cardiovascular and respiratory diseases. They shared the latest developments and successful experiences of global health promotion efforts, and stressed the importance of government leadership, inter-department cooperation and social participation. With an in-depth explanation of the concepts and approaches of promoting the construction of Healthy China, the experts proposed targeted and applicable suggestions for making policies. Their participation has greatly enhanced the academic influence of the forum and helped to strike the accord among all the participants including officials from the administrative departments. The forum will push to form and strengthen the synergy of "Health in All Policies".

Part II

Address

Address

LIU Xu

Chinese Academy of Engineering

Respected President WANG Longde, Respected Deputy Director WANG Guoqiang, Respected Minister SONG Jun, Academicians, friends from home and abroad, ladies and gentlemen,

Good Morning!

Today we gather here to celebrate the inauguration of the International Top-level Forum on Engineering Science and Technology Development Strategy "Healthy China" hosted by Chinese Academy of Engineering. On behalf of the Chinese Academy of Engineering as well as the President Mr. ZHOU Ji, I would like to extend my warm welcome to all the Chinese and foreign friends. And I would like to say a big "Thank You" to Chinese Preventive Medicine Association as well as all the other organizing departments and their staffs.

Health is an eternal topic of mankind. The people's health is an important symbol of national prosperity and strength. Mr. XI Jinping, General Secretary of the Communist Party of China has attached high importance to the people's health. He pointed out clearly that without national health, there will be no all-round well-off society. Healthy China is the goal of new era proposed by the Central Committee of CPC with XI Jinping at its core. In 2015, Healthy China was initiated as national strategy during the fifth plenary session of the 18th CPC Central Committee. The First National Health and Fitness Conference in this new century was held in 2016, with an outcome of *Healthy China 2030 Planning Outline*. In 2017, "to implement Health China strategy" was clearly reaffirmed in the XI Jinping's report at the 19th CPC National Congress. The requirement that "we should improve the national health policy and provide all-round, full-cycle health services to the people" in the new era was put forward. All these fully manifest that our nation has elevated the people's health to unprecedented heights.

Chinese Academy of Engineering is an academic institute with the highest rank of reputation and consultation. It is the think bank of Chinese science and technology. We are hosting this Top-level Forum on "Healthy China" in order to play an active role as thinking bank, enhance the academic lead, closely join and serve the Healthy China strategy. The forum focuses on Healthy China. And we have invited top level experts both home and abroad to have an exchange and discussion on health. They will exchange their views, share their recent progress and advanced ideas so as to reach a wide consensus and make contributions to implementing Healthy China.

This forum has received great attention and support from academicians and experts. 6 academicians from different fields of China will deliver speeches focusing Health in All Policies, from angles of creating health community, promoting health care and improving health policies. They will give an in-depth explanation of the idea and approach to implement Healthy China, as well as share Chinese wisdom and Chinese cases. Several famous foreign experts will brief us about the recent progress and successful experience of international health promotion. They will present us a clear identification of the health indicators under the framework of 2030 sustainable development goals. All these reports will help us fix the concept of "Macro Health", which will definitely play an active role.

Colleagues and friends, around the corner right comes the academic feast. I sincerely hope you will speak out freely and have in-depth discussions, so as to make more contributions to the promotion of Healthy China as well as achieving the goal of national health!

In the end, may I wish this forum a sound success! And I wish all of you good health and good luck! Thank you all!

Part III

Keynote Reports

Strategy as a Priority for the Healthy China Initiative

WANG Longde

Chinese Preventative Medicine Association

Today, I want to have a discussion with you from three perspectives: firstly, I want to probe the domestic and foreign background against which the Healthy China strategy is formulated, so that we can gain a better understanding of the connotation of the strategy; secondly, I want to make a review of the key measures and goals of the Healthy China strategy; and thirdly, I want to make a report on our strategies and experiences in achieving some of the priority goals under the strategy.

First of all, let's take a look at the context in which the Healthy China strategy is formulated. Domestically, years' reform in the health sector has yielded significant benefits, with the health and well-being of the general public improving constantly. However, industrialization, ageing of the population, ecological environment and changes in the lifestyle have all brought about challenges to our health.

Malnutrition and the maternal and neonatal diseases are decreasing significantly, but the risk factors of chronic diseases, like overweight and obesity, are increasing sharply as a major threat to our health. In consequence, the prevalence of chronic diseases is rising fast in our country. Moreover, mortalities attributed to the chronic diseases have accounted for an increasing share of the total deaths due to diseases, to the level of 85% as a matter of fact. In particular, the deaths resulting from cardiovascular diseases cover more than 50% of the total mortalities due to chronic diseases.

The hazard of chronic diseases to human beings is attached with particularly great importance in the international community. The 66th session of General Assembly of the United Nations held a high-level meeting on chronic disease prevention and control in 2011, requiring governments at all levels to formulate multi-agency working guidelines for health issues. The 2030 Agenda for Sustainable Development, adopted by 193 members of the United Nations in 2015, proposed 17 sustainable development goals (SDGs). Almost all of these goals are closely related to health, and particularly, the SDG 2, SDG 3 and SDG 6 set out explicit health-related requirements.

Since 1986, the World Health Organization has been organizing global conferences on health promotion. 8 conferences of that kind have been convened by 2013. Each of the health promotion conferences has proposed some important work to do with respect to health promotion: the 1986 meeting specified the five areas of health promotion; the 1988 conference proposed to formulate health promotion public policies; and the 1991 meeting proposed such important idea as creating health-supportive environment.

The 9th global conference on health promotion was held in Shanghai, with the theme of "Sustainable Development and Health Promotion". It explored how to have health promotion fit with the UN agenda on sustainable development.

In formulating the Healthy China strategy, we have a relatively sounder foundation. In 2008, the then health minister CHEN Zhu proposed a Healthy China 2020 strategic research program with a view to improving the health conditions of both urban and rural residents and the overall health level of nationals. The research program put forward a two-step work guideline and 12 objectives, including mainly the followings: increasing the life expectancy, narrowing regional disparities, developing health industries, and performing governmental functions, etc. In addition, the program made 10 policy recommendations to achieve those objectives to ensure that national health conditions see further improvement.

So in the previous section, I have made a brief introduction to the background for formulation of the Healthy China strategy.

Now with regard to the main content of the Healthy China strategy, I'd like to sum up as follows.

The 5th plenary session of the 18th CPC Central Committee set forth the ambitious Healthy China strategy. Moreover, President XI Jinping clarified the guideline for the health work in the new era in the First National Health and Fitness Conference held in 2016. The biggest difference between the new era guideline and the old ones lies in the fact that it expressly "incorporates health into all policies".

Subsequently, the politburo of the CPC Central Committee adopted the *Healthy China 2030 Planning Outline*. This is actually a program of actions to promote the Healthy China initiative in the 15 years to come. The report of the 19th CPC National

Congress again stressed the need to implement the Healthy China strategy with a view to providing the general public with comprehensive health services throughout their life cycles.

What are the key points of the *Healthy China 2030 Planning Outline* then? First of all, it sets out four principles to be observed in building a Healthy China. There is the principle of regarding health as a priority. There is the principle of making innovation in the health development models to establish systems with Chinese characteristics that promote the health of all people. In addition, there is the principle of following the scientific development concept, that is, to combine prevention and treatment with prevention as a priority and to improve the health services in particular. Finally, there is the principle of fairness and justness, that is, to narrow the gap in health service quality between different population groups. In addition to the principles, the program also stipulates the strategic theme of the Healthy China initiative, including the basic pathway and the fundamental purpose. The basic pathway is through joint development and sharing between the supply and demand sides, while the fundamental purpose is to achieve health in all respects.

The strategic development goals fall into two stages: in terms of the key health indicators, China must be among the best of the medium-to-high income countries by 2020 and among the best of the high income countries by 2030.

The Outline also put forward some concrete indicators. They are 13 indicators to be achieved in five areas, including the increase in expected life expectancy, improvement of health literacy and expansion of the health industry, etc. Here, I'd like to talk about the life expectancy problem.

As we know, previously, we used life expectancy to measure the health level of a country's nationals. However, a big problem facing the mankind today is the fact that we may be able to live long, but may not be able to live healthily and happily. At the beginning of this century, the World Health Organization proposed the new indicator of healthy life expectancy. Subsequently, we can see that the gap between the life expectancy and the healthy life expectancy in the developed countries stood around 10 years. In China, however, we are not yet in a position to measure the healthy life expectancy of all residents. Some regions did have made some local research. For example, Beijing undertook a research on the healthy life expectancy of its residents in 2012 and found that the gap between the life expectancy and the healthy life expectancy is 20 years. A fact is particularly clear. That is, a Beijing resident who is healthy at the age of 18 may not be able to live in healthy status into his sixties. So this is a significant problem in China, a trend for young people to suffer chronic diseases. It is true that we are not yet in a position to measure the healthy life expectancy of all residents across the country, but we can't be like this forever. Can't we create conditions to conduct such measurement at least before 2020? So a new goal in the *Healthy China 2030 Planning Outline* has been set out, that is, to have the healthy life expectancy of all nationals see a significant increase by 2030.

Now I'd like to talk about my understanding about how to achieve priority goals of the Healthy China initiative. Important goals must be accompanied by focused strategies, but to achieve important goals, major problems need to be identified in the first place. What are the major problems in the Healthy China initiative, then? The first is the lack of coordination across the society, for a situation where all government departments and all social communities participate is not yet to be created. Meanwhile, there is the basic problem of low health literacy among our nationals and the high prevalence of chronic diseases, as well as the commonality of such unhealthy behaviors as smoking and drinking to excess. There is also the problem in service provision, for our service system is not well suited to the health needs of our residents. In an era when chronic diseases predominate, participation of the medical organizations is very important. However, an absolute majority of the medical service providers in China are focused on disease diagnosis and treatment, rather than on screening and control of hazardous risks. In this sense, therefore, the chronic disease prevention and control system in China is still in the startup stage, resulting in the extremely low level of control of the cardiovascular diseases, hypertension, dyslipidemia and hyperglycemia, etc.

Now I want to talk about the prevalence of stroke, the first cause of death for our nationals. The study conducted in the last few years proves that nearly 50% of the stroke patients are middle-aged people, whose morbidity and death or disabilities resulting from stroke have extremely severe consequences to their families and the society as a whole. According to forecast of the World Bank, if this situation remains unchanged, the current number of stroke patients, which ranges from 11 million to 12 million, will increase to 31 million in 2030. A further analysis on the age of people highly vulnerable to stroke finds that people in their middle ages account for as many as 60%. This basic condition fits perfectly with the World Bank's forecast. We think that this is one of the most important factors bearing on the health of our nationals. So we submitted a proposal to the Central Committee of the CPC in the capacity of academicians and both the President XI Jinping and Vice Premier LIU Yandong made written comments requiring us to screen and control risk factors of stroke among the middle-aged population.

So what strategies shall we adopt to solve the major problems? We think that actions need to be taken in the following areas: clarifying responsibilities by making laws; laying a sound foundation by improving the health literacy; preventing and controlling hazard risks with priority given to the key factors; creating systems and new models; and undertaking monitoring and supervision to improve effectiveness.

Responsibilities should be clarified first. The central government has set out clear requirements, but how will the requirements be met? First and foremost, the responsibilities of competent ministries of the central government should be clear with a view to establishing a chronic disease prevention and control system at the national level and then including the medical organizations into the system. Next, the central government must specify priorities and goals and guide the work of local governments by setting up demonstration projects. Take the Ministry of Finance for instance. Shouldn't it study and issue policies for government to purchase services? To improve public health, the establishment of a tiered healthcare system is very important. However, the realization of tiered healthcare requires us to improve the quality of medical practitioners at the grassroots and solve the problem in a bottom-up manner. However, the capacity to provide services at the grassroots is lacking at the moment. So it is necessary for medical experts at higher levels to provide training locally. If this is really the case, however, who will fund the training? The current approach is to make training assignments to hospitals and have them fund the training all by themselves. This approach is not sustainable, in fact. So how should the government take on the funding responsibility? In the past, you were qualified as a clinical practitioner if you were good at diagnosing and treating diseases. In the era of epidemic chronic diseases, you are no longer so if you are good at those skills only, because every clinical practitioner must have the knowledge and skills necessary to prevent and control major chronic diseases and actually do so on their respective posts. On the other hand, if we are to improve the health literacy of our nationals, then the communication department is a very important area of work. How can we mobilize the communication departments to put the publicity of health science and knowledge high on their work agendas? This certainly requires funding support on the part of government.

Regarding the medical insurance authorities, the current policy they practice is to reimburse expenses for treatment and life-saving rescues in particular after diseases have occurred and seldom reimburse expenses incurred in the efforts to control risk factors of chronic diseases. In the developed countries, however, people with mere chronic risk factors, like overweight and obesity, and even exercise activities, have been covered by medical insurance. So shouldn't we review our concerned policies?

In order to improve the health literacy, we must start from educating children at a young age and even educating their parents at the same time, so that our children can fall into healthy lifestyles and habits during their childhood. In this regard, the education sector must take on the responsibility, which is unshirkable to them. In addition, the civil service authorities must not only do the practice of just issuing certificates of marriage; in fact, they can go further to provide education on the knowledge of having a healthy baby and scientific ways of raising children for young men and women who apply to them for marriage registration. It is no doubt that all the newly wedded people hope to give birth to a healthy child and have a child who grows healthily.

I remember that many enterprises and other organizations had medical clinic two to three decades ago, but these medical facilities have all disappeared nowadays. All members of the functional community end up visiting provincial or city medical organizations when they are ill, placing an unbearable burden on the latter. Do our workers take physical examinations? Are the major risk factors threatening their health discovered? How are the canteens of employers doing in providing healthy food? Are they feeding workers with high salt, high sugar and high fat food? Is it necessary for employers to designate personnel to take charge of such affairs? Can the social groups, like women's federations, do some training on healthy diet? Women play a very important role in family life, so much so that their family members eat whatever they cook. If they provide healthy food, then the health of their whole family will be ensured. Presently, we are trying to include such safeguards of health into the health law being made in an effort to ensure that the principle of "Health in All Policies" is put in place.

If we can improve the health literacy, then we can lay a solid foundation for the Healthy China initiative. Analyses of the World Health Organization on global researchers have found that lifestyles and behaviors have a 60% impact on lifespan and health. However, the health literacy of ours is very low today, with only one out of ten people having the basic health literacy. So if this situation remains, it is impossible for us to put the prevalence of chronic diseases under control.

Then, there is the need to prevent and control risk factors and give priority to the key ones. Some risk factors, like hypertension, are major threats to our health. The United States has summed up its experience in reducing the level of morbidity and mortality due to stroke in the past five decades or so and finds that the control of blood pressure, blood fat, blood glucose and smoking, and the control of blood pressure in particular, is the key to such reduction, so much so that if the blood pressure is well controlled, then nearly half of the stroke cases can be prevented. In China, however, the level of awareness, control and treatment of hypertension is still very low. Many rural residents have never taken their blood pressure; many hypertension patients have never taken any medicines, unaware of the huge risks from high blood pressure. These years, we have taken some measures in this respect, including mobilizing 318 provincial and municipal hospitals to take part in our stroke prevention and control campaign. These hospitals have gathered more than 1000 county hospitals as assisting organizations, which in turn have secured more than 2700 community or township-level health organizations to engage in the screening and control of stroke. In this campaign, we have worked out a stroke prevention and control strategy, which is described as follows: finding risk factors and giving intervention have the priority; focusing on the grassroots; improving health literacy; giving priority to education and communication; conducting multi-disciplinary cooperation; practicing standardized prevention and control; screening out the high risk population groups; and making targeted interventions.

In that campaign, we have produced teaching materials to promote appropriate medical techniques. In the past few years, we selected 20 provincial and municipal hospitals as the training centers have trained 110000 medical personnels, to which we have communicated some appropriate techniques. For example, severe carotid stenosis is one of the important causes of stroke, but we only performed as many as 247 operations for such patients in 2010. We have focused on promoting such prevention and control technique as the CEA operation in recent years, and performed more than 3000 operations of this kind in each of the past few years. The usage rate of thrombolysis among the stroke patients is as high as 20% – 30% in the developed countries, but is lower than 2% in China. In fact, a majority of the 3A hospitals have not yet made good use of thrombolysis, not to mention the county-level medical providers, so the disability rate is very high among our stroke patients. Theoretically, a hospital with CT scanner is able to do thrombolysis. Moreover, all the hospitals at the county level or over have CT scanner, but the technique has not been promoted in the past. In recent years, however, we have exerted great efforts to promote the technique. Previously, patients had to spend two hours doing thrombolysis even in provincial or city hospitals, while the international requirement is in one hour. So we have been reforming our service procedures, limiting the time spent on each stage of thrombolysis. If you spend more time than required, you are not qualified. Nowadays, many hospitals designated as stroke prevention and control bases have been able to shorten the time used in thrombolysis to the one hour limit.

In the next step, the priority of our work is to create a one-hour emergency rescue circle for stroke patients and to establish a regional prevention and control network. Via the national prevention and control network and projects, we can screen only a million people over the age of 40 every year, so when will the general public benefit from it? This is why the national prevention and control program expressly set out the plan to create a regional prevention and control network for stroke. The network must be established before 2020. The one-hour emergency rescue circle must be set up, too.

There is another system to be established. It is the health education system. The establishment of that system is impossible through only the efforts of the health sector; it requires coordination with the radio, film and television, communication and education sectors. President XI also proposed to create a sound health education system that disseminates health knowledge in a way that is reachable, comprehensible and acceptable to the general public.

Finally, there is the need to undertake supervision to improve effectiveness. In the past, we failed to fulfill some principles set out by the central government just because of the lack of supervision and inspection. So the *Healthy China 2030 Planning Outline* has laid down explicit requirements for monitoring, evaluation and supervision.

I believe that if we can really put in place the guideline of incorporating health into all policies under the work mechanism featuring government leadership, multi-agency cooperation and social participation, we can definitely and effectively muster all social forces to achieve the goal of building a Healthy China as early as possible.

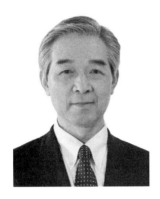 **WANG Longde** is Academician of the Chinese Academy of Engineering, is concurrently President of the Chinese Preventive Medicine Association, Member of the Standing Committee of the 12th National People's Congress and Vice Chairman of the Education, Science, Culture and Public Health Committee of the National People's Congress. Previously, he was Deputy Party Chief and Vice Minister of the Ministry of Health. His part-time positions include Director of the Disease Prevention and Control Experts Committee, National Health and Family Planning Commission; Director of the Health Promotion and Education Experts Committee; Deputy Director of the Stroke Screening, Prevention and Control Committee; Advisor for Scientific and Technological Innovation Strategies, etc.

He is long engaged in public health administration and academic research in epidemiology and public health promotion. He proposed and actually led the efforts to create an online system for medical providers across the country to directly report infectious diseases and public health emergencies. He researched and then proposed a new strategy to control schistosomiasis that focuses on controlling the sources of infection. He also proposed and organized the national stroke screening, prevention and control project. He has published more than a hundred academic papers in domestic and foreign journals, including the *New England Journal of Medicine*, and has been Editor-in-Chief for several monographs. His honors include the National Science and Technology Progress Award (level 2), the UNAIDS Award for Excellent Leadership and Contribution in Dealing with AIDS, the WHO Stop TB Partnership Kochon Prize, and the WHO World No-tobacco Day Award, etc.

Agriculture, Food Development and National Nutritional Health

LIU Xu

Chinese Academy of Engineering

Today, I'd like to discuss the topic "Agriculture, Food Development and National Nutritional Health" with you from four perspectives: the status quo of agricultural production and food supply in China; the characteristics and trends of residents' food consumption; the status of residents' nutrition and health; and the proposals to develop agriculture and improve the nutritional health of nationals.

The first part of my speech concerns the status quo of agricultural production and food supply in China.

The status quo of agricultural production in China can be summarized as follows. In the first place, the production of various edible farm products is abundant and stable. In 2016, the food production of China weighed 616 million tons, including 207 million tons of rice, 129 million tons of wheat and 220 million tons of maize, down by 0.8% over 2015, resulting in the first decline after 12 consecutive years' increase in the food production. In the same year, the total production of animal products stood at 221 million tons, including 85.40 million tons of meat, 30.95 million tons of eggs, 36.02 million tons of milk, and 69 million tons of aquatic products, standing basically at the same level as in 2015. Still in 2016, the total production of vegetables and fruits exceeded 1 billion tons, parallelled with that of 2015.

In the second place, the conditions of agricultural production have gradual improvements. In 2015, the total power of agricultural machinery reached 1.1 billion kilowatts, with the level of tilling, planting and harvesting mechanization standing at 63%. The mechanization process was particularly fast on the weak links of production of some major crops. In 2015, the level of mechanization for rice planting and maize harvesting exceeded 40% and 63% respectively, up by 19 and 37 percentage points over the end of the 11th Five-Year Plan period. In the same year, the work to identify permanent basic farmland has been conducted on a full scale in the decreasing order of the size of towns, of the proximity to the towns and of the quality of the land, etc., with positive progress already achieved in 106 key cities. Moreover, the social service provision of agricultural machinery has developed in depth from the tilling, planting and harvesting processes to the entire production cycle including the pre-, mid- and post-production processes. With more than 56500 professional agricultural cooperatives, the capacity to provide lifecycle mechanized services has been significantly increased.

In the third place, the food processing capacity has seen fast growth. Since onset of the reform and opening-up drive, the production of the agricultural product processing industry has been growing at an annual average pace of more than 13%, significantly higher than that of the GDP growth in the same period. By 2014, there have been 455000 farm product processing enterprises in China, including 76000 businesses in or over the size designated for statistical purposes. These enterprises have generated 18.48 trillion yuan in prime operating revenue and 1.22 trillion yuan in profit, raising the ratio of the production of the farm product processing industry to the production of agriculture as a whole to 2.1 to 1. Moreover, a development pattern characterized by industry clusters has gradually taken shape, with priority given to grain and oil, meat, dairy product, fruits and vegetables and specialty food. The market shares of emerging convenient food, leisure food and green food are continuing to expand. And the functional food, such as prepared food and health preservation food, is increasingly accepted by consumers.

The general situation of domestic agriculture and of the effective food supply in particular can be described as follows. In terms of the quality assurance, namely, the guarantee of food safety, the quality and safety of food supply in our country has been improving steadily as the overall capacity of agricultural production increases and the opening-up drive steps up in the agricultural sector. For years on end, the overall qualification rate of edible farm products has remained at the level of 96% or over in spot check, keeping the general trend of being stable and changing for better. Throughout the year of 2015, the overall quality compliance rate of farm products stood at 97.1%, with that of vegetables, fruits, tea, livestock and poultry products, and aquatic products standing at 96.1%, 95.6%, 97.6%, 99.4% and 95.5% respectively. In the same year, the area of land subject to environmental monitoring in regions producing green food reached 260 million mu, roughly 4.5 times that of 2000. In terms of the quantity of food supply, namely, the guarantee of availability and quality, the current production and effective supply of food in China is able to meet the consumer demand for nutrition. Given the total food supply level in 2015 and with the lost and inedible part deducted, the food production of China was able to provide 2855 kilocalorie heat, 103 grams protein and 77 grams fat on a per capita basis, which was close to the level in developed countries respectively. On the other hand, the per capita demand of Chinese people for heat, protein and fat is 1910 kilocalorie, 67 grams and 58 grams respectively. From the perspective of the three major nutritional elements, the production and effective supply of food in China is able to meet the healthy demand of domestic residents for nutrition. In terms of the balance between food supply and food demand, the level of food self-sufficiency is on the high side in China, generally speaking, with excessive supply coexisting with short supply in general and standing out for some products in particular. This is the main reason for us to make urgent structural adjustment on the supply side at present and for a foreseeable period in the future.

The second part of my speech concerns the characteristics and trends of residents' food consumption. From the food structure's point of view, the trend of food consumption of Chinese residents over the past three decades finds expression in three respects as follows.

Firstly, the per capita consumption of grains is on the decline, with that of urban residents showing a relatively higher level of stability. Since 1981, the per capita consumption of grains (raw) has generally been decreasing for both urban and rural residents, with that of the urban residents falling from 201 kg to 139 kg in 2009 and remaining stable subsequently and that of the rural residents falling from 260 kg to 176 kg.

Secondly, the per capita consumption of animal products is increasing, but there is still a relatively huge gap between the consumption of urban and rural residents. In the period from 1981 to 2015, the per capita consumption of animal products (in their raw form) of both urban and rural residents has increased, with that of the urban residents growing from 37.1 kg to 106.1 kg and that of the rural residents from 12.2 kg to 57.5 kg respectively. So the absolute gap in such consumption is widening, but the relative gap is narrowing, with the ratio of the urban consumption to the rural consumption dropping from 3 : 1 to 1.8 : 1.

Thirdly，the per capita consumption of vegetables is decreasing overall，but the reduction on the part of urban residents is relatively small. In the period from 1981 to 2015，the per capita consumption by rural residents dropped from 126.0 kg to 98.1 kg，down by about 1/5，while that of the urban residents dropped from 152.3 kg to 139.3 kg，with the reduction less than 10%.

Now I'd like to make a judgment with respect to the overall trend of food consumption in the future China. Currently，the Engel coefficient of the urban and rural residents in China has downed to 36.2% and 39.3% respectively. According to the standard issued by the FAO，China has now entered into a relatively affluent stage of the socio-economic development. Given the experience of regions with similar consumption patterns，when the Engel coefficient of residents ranges from 20% to 40%，the dietary structure of Chinese residents will see a prominent upgrading process in the future，that is，the consumption of grains will decrease；the consumption of animal products will increase slightly；and the total food demand will increase slowly.

The third part of my speech is about the status of residents' nutrition and health.

An analysis of the nutrition intake will find that：firstly，the caloric intake of Chinese nationals has gradually declined over the past 30 years or so；secondly，the intake of proteins has been stable in general；thirdly，the share of animal proteins in the total protein intake has significantly risen；and fourthly，the intake of fat has been on the rise overall，which is a major cause of the high prevalence of nutrition-related diseases，such as obesity.

Regarding the health conditions of our nationals，firstly，the rate of growth retardation among children and youths has fallen. Compared with 2002，the growth retardation rate of children and youths aged 6 to 17 during the period of 2010−2012 has fallen by 3.1 percentage points，a reduction of 49%. Secondly，the prevalence of anemia among various population groups has significantly fallen，too. Compared with 2002, the prevalence of anemia among urban and rural population groups，including both sexes and all age brackets，has dropped sharply from 2010 to 2012，with that of rural residents falling more sharply，relatively speaking. Thirdly，the number of overweight and obese adults has been increasing constantly. Across the country，the proportion of overweight and obese adults stands at 30% and 12% respectively，up by 18 and 8 percentage points over 1992. Fourthly，the prevalence of diabetes among adults has risen explosively to 9.7%，more than twice that of 2002.

As the saying goes, "food is of primal importance to the people". It is an important material basis for human beings to live, grow and stay healthy, bearing on the quality of nationals and socio-economic development. Eating one's fill, eating up to the standard and eating in a healthy manner are important preconditions for health preservation, but health is subject to multiple factors, including heredity, psychology, ecological environment and market competition, etc. This is the main reason why the government has one after another issued *Healthy China 2030 Planning Outline*, *National Nutrition Plan (2017–2030)* and *China Food and Nutrition Development Outline (2014–2020)*, etc.

Healthy China 2030 Planning Outline stressed "the need to incorporate health into all policies, accelerate transforming the pattern of development for the health sector, maintain and protect public health in an all-rounded manner and throughout lifecycles and improve the health conditions and health equality significantly, with improvement of the public health as the core goal, reform and innovation of systems and mechanisms as the driving force and popularization of healthy lifestyles, optimization of health services, perfection of health insurance, creation of healthy environment and development of health industries as the top priorities". Meanwhile, the Outline highlighted the need to "formulate and implement national nutrition plan", "promote healthy lifestyles" and regard the effort to "guide a reasonable diet" as a primary measure to "shape autonomous and self-disciplined health behaviors".

National Nutrition Plan (2017–2030) emphasized that we must take a down-to-earth and forward-looking approach to the nutritional health of our nationals throughout their life cycles and health processes, taking public health as the core, giving priority to popularization of nutritional health knowledge, optimization of nutritional health services, perfection of nutritional health systems, creation of nutritional health environment and development of nutritional health industries and incorporating nutrition into all health policies, with a view to meeting the public need for nutritional health, improving the health conditions of all people and laying a solid foundation for the effort to build a Healthy China.

China Food and Nutrition Development Outline (2014–2020) stated emphatically that, on the one hand, the food and nutrition development in China has scored significant achievements in recent years, as illustrated by the steady expansion of the comprehensive production capacity, the basic balance between food supply and demand, the stability and even improvement of food safety in general, and the significant improvement of residents' nutritional health conditions, but on the other hand, there are still problems that require great attention, such as the inability to cater to the nutritional needs, the prominent coexistence of nutrition deficiency and nutrition excess, the imperative task to ensure basic nutrition for tens of millions of poverty-stricken people and low-income people and the serious lack of nutrition and health-related knowledge, etc.

In the report of the 19th National Congress of the Communist Party of China (CPC), General Secretary XI Jinping underlined the necessity to win the battle against poverty, that is, to ensure that all the rural poor under the existing poverty criteria are out of poverty, all poverty-stricken counties are relieved of poverty, and the regional poverty problem is solved by 2020, assisting those who are really poor and making real efforts to relieve poverty. Moreover, there are the needs to implement the rural revitalization strategy, to ensure national food safety so that food is in our own hand, and to practice the Healthy China strategy. As health is an important indicator of national prosperity and state power, there is the need to undertake the patriotic health campaign, promote healthy and civilized lifestyles and prevent and control major diseases while focusing on prevention. In addition, the food safety strategy must be executed, too to reassure the general public with respect to what they eat.

In the fourth part, I'd like to explore recommendations concerning agricultural development and improvement of the national nutrition and health conditions. To do so, I will focus on three aspects: the agricultural supply side, the demand side and the macro-control measures.

On the agricultural supply side, there remains the need to increase the total supply and improve the quality of food. Firstly, the food production has to be increased. According to the forecast on food demand due to population growth, the total population of China will stand at 1.5 billion or so, the annual per capita food consumption will reach 450–470 kg and the total food consumption will amount to 700 million tons or so by 2035 when China basically achieves modernization. That's to say, the food production must increase by nearly 100 million tons to meet the consumer demand. Secondly, there is the need to adjust the agricultural structure to raise the proportion of quality products and the need to implement the food-to-feed reform to increase the share of premium Japonica rice, high/low-gluten wheat, and silage maize, etc., with a view to ensuring that domestic production matches demand in terms of both quantity and quality. Thirdly, there is the need to improve the quality of food by accelerating development, application and promotion of high quality animal and plant germplasm resources, upgrading the crude workshop-style processing techniques of traditional farm products, and improving the quality and nutritional functions of edible farm products. Fourthly, there is the need to develop nutrition-enhanced products. Research shows that the mere intake of nutrition from food is more often than not insufficient to meet the needs of human bodies. So it has become a new normal to supplement the health needs with the intake of dietary supplements and nutrition-enhanced food.

On the demand side, there is the need to promote implementation of the dietary guidelines, add some new consumer subsidy and food assistance and provide monitoring and guidance for food consumption. Firstly, efforts must be made to promote implementation of the 2016 Dietary Guidelines for Chinese Residents. For this purpose, the mainstream media, like TV and internet, must be used as primary channels to disseminate knowledge on diet and nutrition. In addition, it is advisable to borrow the foreign practice of levying consumption tax against high sugar and high fat food, with the tax collected to be used for the purpose of improving public health facilities. It is also desirable to advance the salt and edible oil reduction initiatives and the sugar and alcohol control campaigns across the country to shield consumers from the detrimental effect of unhealthy food. Moreover, subsidies can be employed to lower the prices of fresh fruits and vegetables by 10%–30% in an effort to encourage the consumption of fruits and vegetables. Important biofortification projects should also be established to increase support for research, development and industrialization of biofortified products blessed with high quality, high yield and high adaptability. Secondly, food assistance must be provided for poverty-stricken and low income groups. Food consumption is both an economic and social problem. Even in highly food-sufficient countries, there is still the problem of food safety and supply concerning the vulnerable low income minorities. According to the rural poverty line of 2300 yuan (at the 2010 constant price) per capita per annum, there are still as many as 43.35 million poor rural residents in China by 2016, who suffer from inadequate dietary intake and lack of micro nutrients. So it is recommended that the government distribute food coupons as soon as possible and provide free lunch for primary and secondary schools in remote, poverty-stricken regions to meet the basic need for nutrition of the poor and low income population groups and primary and secondary students. It is also recommended to promote nutrition-sensitive agriculture and particularly develop distinctive, premium food resources and produce new food materials in the poverty-stricken areas. Thirdly, food consumption monitoring and guiding platforms must be established. For this purpose, efforts must be made to create county-based monitoring stations integrating monitoring of both food production and consumption with nutrition education. Computer networks and mobile communication platforms must be used as online evaluation tools to support self-evaluation of dietary quality on the part of residents. Individualized nutrition recipes and nutrition supplement plans must be designed for key population groups. Factors affecting residents' food consumption should also be studied to propose targeted policies for consumption guidance and nutrition intervention.

At the macro-control level, governments at all levels must strengthen their guidance and commitment to the food nutrition work. Firstly, food nutrition-related legislation must be accelerated to promote legitimate management of food and nutrition. The nutrition intervention against key territories and population groups, the strengthening of nutrition and health guidance for schools, kindergartens and the elderly care facilities and the ensuring of the basic nutrition needs for the low income groups must be regarded as responsibilities of governments at all levels and their affiliated departments in nutrition promotion and intervention. Secondly, the *National Nutrition Plan* (*2017 –2030*) must be put in place to create a coordination mechanism involving agricultural, health, education, science and technology, and poverty relief authorities and to advance the food and nutrition cause. Thirdly, residents' nutrition security must be included into the national 13th Five-Year Plan as a development goal. Based on local resources and consumption patterns, dietary models for different regions and different population groups can be created. Moreover, the food nutrition and health conditions of residents can be incorporated as a performance indicator for local governments.

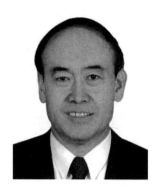

LIU Xu is Academician of the CAE, the Former Vice President of the CAE, the Crop Germplasm Resources Scientist, and the Former Vice President of Chinese Academy of Agricultural Sciencess.

Following the Law of Brain Development to Foster Healthy and Excellent Future Generations

WEI Yu

Chinese Academy of Engineering

General Secretary XI Jinping attaches extremely great importance to the development and education of children in the poverty-stricken areas, pointing out that "education must precede poverty relief" and stressing the need to "prevent intergenerational transfer of poverty". In 2016, six ministries and commissions of the central government, represented by the Ministry of Education and the National Development and Reform Commission, jointly issued China's first ever five-year plan for poverty alleviation through education. Subsequently, effective measures have been taken in that regard and great progress have been made so far in carrying out the poverty alleviation through education and delivering the principle of education equality. The report to the 19th CPC National Congress set forth the new concept of "children's right to good care" for the first time. Inspired by the spirit of the 19th CPC National Congress, we are expected to do a better job in precision poverty relief by resorting to the power of science and technology.

Nowadays, we all think highly of the health conditions of our nationals and of the importance of disease prevention. However, health is not just the well-being of the body, like heart, lung and liver, etc. It should also take into account the well-being of the brain and the mental part of the human being. To some extent, it is safe to say that the health of brain is even more important than that of the body, because what identifies you as you and as a human being is exactly your unique and powerful brain.

A definition of health has been given in the charter of the World Health Organization in 1946 when it was founded.

"Health is a state of complete physical, mental and social well-being and not merely the absence of disease or infirmity."

The definition has different Chinese translations. Both emphasize that health is not just the physical well-being; and that it should also include the mental and social well-being of a human being. As a matter of fact, this is often overlooked and even forgotten by us.

So when it comes to health and the prevention of diseases, we can say that education and healthcare are the two integral parts of them. The first and foremost is science education in schools, which is an effective way to disseminate knowledge of disease prevention and health and sanitation. But today, I would like to focus on integrated projects aimed at assisting children in adversity. Some content has already been addressed in several WeChat articles previously published, so I will not repeat that. Instead, I will add the mechanism for adversity to be embedded into the biological system.

All adversities, not just physical and sexual abuse, but even the lack of appropriate parenting environment, like neglect, apathy and overburden from study, will do harm to children. The basic mechanism is that the stress (typically known as psychological pressure) will trigger a stress response on the part of the human body and make the HPA axle generate hormones of the cortisone type. For all abuses that do harm to the development of children, the key is the enduring harm they do to the stress response of the HPA axle.

In a bid to protect himself, man has retained and developed his ability to make response to external stimulus in the process of evolution. The threatening stimulus from outside will be transmitted to the brain via the sensory system, then through the hypothalamus and to the different regions of the brain, immediately triggering a series of physical responses, including the automatically activated sympathetic nervous system, the endocrine system, the metabolic system and the immune system, etc. Of them, the HPA axle is the key. In response to a threat, the HPA axle will be activated at once and man will make response immediately along the route from hypothalamus to the pituitary and then to the adrenals. The hypothalamus will release CRH; the CRH will in turn stimulate the pituitary to produce ACTH; and the ACTH will then stimulate the periphery of the adrenals, namely, the adrenal cortex, to make CORT. The CORT then enters into the blood circulation system, changing the vegetative nervous system and the hormone system quickly, elevating the blood sugar content to provide more energy for combat and/or escape, and adjusting the state of the body, such as heart rate, breathing and the muscle strength, for the purpose of making response to the external threat.

The stress response feature of the HPA axle and the CORT's capacity to regulate the ACTH and CRH is related to the level of activation of the brain regions concerned. The HPA axle will be activated in a response to stress. But when the stress recedes, the feedback loops at different levels of the stress system will be activated to terminate the response of the HPA axle, returning the body to the original state of balance. Such regulatory function is partly achieved through two types of cortisone receptors, which are mainly the GR and the MR. These receptors will combine with the cortisone molecules and initiate a series of processes on the genetic level, thereby regulating the expression many different genes. This is actually the study of the epigenomics. GR and MR not only exist in the HPA axle system, but also exist in many brain regions, like the hippocampus and the frontal cortex. Moreover, GR is almost ubiquitous in all the cells of the body. This is why changes in the level of cortisone will affect the functioning of many organs. The hippocampus and the frontal cortex are important brain regions that regulate the HPA axle and enable it to return to balance and therefore achieve the negative feedback. Another is the amygdaloid body, which is called the "engine of emotions". In contrast to the hippocampus, the amygdaloid body functions to make positive feedback, activating and aggravating the stress response. When the stress is removed, the frontal cortex will return the amygdaloid body to the original normal state of balance.

So the reason why the HPA axle is retained in the process of evaluation is that it is beneficial to the survival of the mankind as a positive mechanism. However, if the stress response is excessive and enduring, it will lead to harmful consequences.

According to the effect of stress response, we can divide the stress response into three types.

(1) Positive Stress Response. This is a normal physical response. It is even necessary for us to promote children's development on some occasions, such as the first time for a child to meet with his new carer, the presence of emotions in the process of learning, and the occasion of prophylactic inoculation, etc. In the presence of positive emotions in learning, the memory will be enhanced. The main characteristic of a positive stress response is the heightened heart rate and the somewhat increase in the cortisone hormone produced. When the stress disappears, the body will return to normal, a state of dynamic balance.

（2）Tolerable Stress Response. Confronted with considerable stimulus or strike，such as unexpected assault，encounter with dangerous animals，occurrence of natural disasters or loss of loved ones，human beings will experience stress response. If the stress lasts relatively a short time，especially when the carers play a supportive or mitigating role on the side of the affect child to help him/her adapt to such impact，then the body of the affected child will remain resilient. When the stress disappears，the brain and other organs of the body can simply recover from the harm done to them.

（3）Toxic Stress Response. If a child suffers severe，frequent or long-lasting harm and lack necessary support from his/her carers，then the HPA axle will stay in the state of stress response continuously. This will make the concentration of cortisone remain at an abnormally high level，change the genetic expression of the GR and MR，reduce the child's regulatory ability to recover balance and alter the HPA axle's response threshold. Meanwhile，as the cortisone circulates across the body，it will damage the structure of the brain and affect the normal functions of many other organs.

The hippocampus brain region，as shown in the picture，plays a very important role in the learning process. It is where the declarative memory takes shape and therefore has a direct bearing on the development of human intelligence. When the body experiences a stress response，it will identify the nature of the stress and generate negative feedback to help the HPA axle recover original balance. In a toxic stress response，however，cortisone will impair the functions of the hippocampal neural cells，weaken the HPA axle's capacity to reinstate balance and reduce children's memory and learning ability. For some children who have experienced adversities during pregnancy or in their early childhood，the hippocampus region tends to be smaller than that of the normal children. Similarly，the development of the frontal cortex，which is also responsible for generating negative feedback，controlling the stress response and helping the body and the brain recover balance，will be obstructed. Moreover，the link between the prefrontal cortex and the amygdaloid body will be weakened，too，resulting in the impairment of the ability to regulate emotions. Conversely，a toxic stress response tends to make the amygdaloid body bigger than normal and more sensitive to external stimulus. So an enduring high concentration of the cortisone will reduce the systemic ability of the human body to reinstate the HPA axle into balance，elevate the response threshold of the HPA axle and undermine the control of cognitive and emotional processes.

Pregnancy and early childhood are both periods when the HPA axle is most shapable. During pregnancy, whether because the mother suffers mental disorders such as depression and anxiety or because she abuses or misuses drugs, the fetus will be adversely affected if the mother therefore experiences a toxic stress response. After birth into the early childhood, if the child suffers toxic stress response himself/herself, the damage done will be aggravated. It will not only affect development of the infant, but also bear on the health and behavior of the child throughout his/her life, by increasing his/her susceptibility to stress response-related diseases and generating risks of cognitive disorder, mental illness, and such misconduct as drug abuse, suicide and violence, etc. Nelson et al. has also proven the foregoing mechanism true through their empirical research on the children in Romanian orphanages.

In recent years, scientists have also studied the interrelations between the intestinal microflora and the brain, which play also via the HPA axle in a large part.

According to the solid evidence provided by scientific research, the WHO, the UNICEF and the World Bank, among other international organizations, have been calling on national governments and concerned parties to realize the fact that the key to the human sustainable development lies in the development of the mankind itself and the need to take a serious look at how to effectively eradicate such problems as poverty and socio-economic inequality. They also call on countries to put the results of scientific research into practice and implement integrated assistance projects by combining the nutrition project for disadvantaged children with the projects aimed at promoting children's development in their early childhood.

Overall, ① scientific research tells us that the 1000 day period from conception to the 2-3 years after birth is an important period for human development. It is both a period of opportunity to promote lifelong development and a sensitive period when adverse conditions (poverty, abuse, neglect, etc.) have serious negative effect on children. ② The adversities in the early childhood will substantially be embedded into children's biosystem and alter their biological conditions and development. They will affect the health of the victimized children for a life time, reduce their cognitive competence and undermine their capacity to control their behaviors and emotions, resulting in the occurrence of addition, suicide and a variety of anti-social behaviors. ③ The harms done to the affected children may be transferred to their offspring through their behaviors after they become parents as well as through different epigenetic mechanisms. ④ The most effective way to avoid and make up for such adverse effect is to provide the underprivileged children with ongoing, supportive family parenting environment.

Therefore, it is recommended that the government shift the point of time for poverty alleviation to the earliest 1000 day period of a life and implement integrated assistance initiatives for children by integrating the health, education and other forces to support and improve the parenting quality of children living in difficulty. This is an effective measure to enhance the precision of poverty alleviation, achieve education equality and stop intergeneration transfer of poverty. It is a matter of great importance that bears on the sustainable development of the Chinese nation.

Education needs to follow the law of education development. Education is actually to build the brain of children, so it must follow the law of the brain development, too, with a view to making our children become excellent and healthy constructors and successors.

Education in compliance with the law of development and deep integration of information technologies are both important indicators of education modernization.

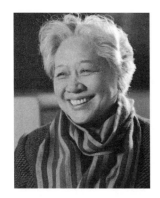

WEI Yu   is Academician of CAE, Member of the China National Education Advisory Committee, Vice Chairman of Chinese Society for Cognitive Science, Member of *MBE* editorial board, Member of the IAP-IBSE council, Former President of Southeast University, Former Vice Minister of Education Ministry, Former Vice President of China Association for Science and Technology.

Better Nutrition for a Healthy China

CHEN Junshi

China National Center for Food Safety Risk Assessment

Today, I would like to talk about the *National Nutrition Plan (2017-2030)*. But I do not want to spend too much time talking about the content, as this document can be downloaded online. The key point I want to make is about the background. Why the *National Nutrition Plan 2017-2030* is issued and why it is issued by the State Council?

In 2012, the World Health Organization (WHO) released the Global Nutrition Targets 2025. In 2014, the Second International Conference on Nutrition was held in Rome, jointly organized by WHO and the Food and Agriculture Organization of the United Nations (FAO) with delegations from 150 countries participated. It is not an ordinary academic exchange but an intergovernmental conference. The Conference, for the first time, defined malnutrition internationally. We often said in China that "we are now facing the dual burden of undernutrition and overnutrition", which is not scientific and precise enough, as defined by the Conference. Malnutrition, by definition, includes the following three forms:

The first is undernutrition, or put it simple, "not having enough to eat". In terms of nutrition, it means protein energy deficiency.

The second is micronutrient deficiencies, or in a more common way, "hidden hunger", which means that one seems full, but has inadequate intake of vitamins and minerals. So it is called micronutrient deficiencies.

The third is overweight and obesity. This is a big change from the traditional concept, and provides a standardized expression. At present, overweight and obesity are collectively classified as one of the three major forms of malnutrition. In China, it means "imbalance of eating and exercise".

Comparing the three forms of malnutrition with the current situation and existing problems in China, we can see that: first, we met over a billion people's basic needs. In other words, we have enough to eat, or at least, we basically have adequate food. There are, of course, very few people who are hungry. But regarding the 1.3 billion people in the country, having enough food to eat has been basically realized. Research shows that dietary energy intake has been relatively adequate since 1982, per capita energy intake reaching or even exceeding the recommended amount.

The second is stunted growth of children and adolescents. We can see that the national growth retardation rate which was 4.7% in 2012, has been greatly improved in recent decades. However, according to the survey results of Nutrition Improvement Plan for Rural Compulsory Education Students, there are still some gaps between the poverty-stricken areas and the national average. The growth retardation rates of these areas in 2013 and 2014 were 8.0% and 7.5% respectively.

Third, the most important problem of malnutrition is micronutrient deficiencies, in particular iron deficiency which will cause iron deficiency anemia. Although the overall anemia prevalence in the past two decades has been declined significantly, it is still high among three key populations, especially among children aged 12 – 24 months and pregnant women, with an anemic prevalence of about 16%. This problem in elderly people aged 75 and above is also serious, with a higher anemia prevalence than children and pregnant women.

Fourth, overweight and obesity are major nutritional problems in our country. Many chronic diseases, as Academician WANG Longde just mentioned in his report, are commonly caused by overweight and obesity.

Under such circumstances, the best policy era in nutrition and health is ushered in 2016 and 2017. To solve these nutritional problems, the government should introduce policies that not only refer to China's policies but also international policies. At present, the *United Nations Sustainable Development Goals* (SDGs) is the largest international policy documents. Among the Goals, the SDG 2 refers to "end all forms of malnutrition", and SDG 3 refers to health, infectious diseases, chronic non-communicable diseases and emergencies of women and children. To achieve these goals, nutrition is an important measure. Generally speaking, with improved nutrition, SDG 2 and SDG 3 are much easier to achieve; otherwise, they are difficult or even impossible to achieve.

The 17 SDGs have a very long list. Besides SDG 2 and SDG 3, nutrition is the enabler of all other Goals, which means that nutrition enables the accomplishment of all

SDGs. In summary, SDGs' vision of nutrition is to end malnutrition in all its forms and to meet the nutritional needs for the full life cycle, including the first 1000 days of life, as well as to provide necessary global nutrition actions for safe, healthy and sustainable food.

In 2014, General Secretary XI Jinping pointed out that: "the all-round moderately prosperous society could not be achieved without people's all-round health." In 2016, "promoting a healthy China" was clearly stated in the 13th Five-Year Plan. In the same year, a national meeting on health was held and the *Healthy China 2030 Planning Outline* was released in October.

The *Healthy China 2030 Planning Outline* is a guiding policy document issued by the state. I would like to emphasize that without improved nutrition, most indicators will certainly not be completed. So the importance of nutrition is obvious. Moreover, there is one single section called "guiding healthy dietary" in *Healthy China 2030 Planning Outline*, and the first half sentence of this section is formulating and implementing the *National Nutrition Plan*. *Healthy China 2030 Planning Outline* was issued in October last year and at that time, the work was underway to develop the *National Nutrition Plan*. Vice Premier LIU Yandong foresightedly directed the National Health and Family Planning Commission to take the lead in drafting the *National Nutrition Plan*, at that time called the *National Nutrition Improvement Action Plan*. Vice Premier LIU Yandong's instruction is very brief with only two points. The first is to combine with disease prevention and treatment, in particular, chronic diseases. The second is to boost the development of the food industry.

The drafting of the *National Nutrition Plan* started in February, 2016. And the Plan was issued by the State Council on July 13, 2017, just one and a half years later. It was highly efficient. As one of the experts who had undergone the entire process, I deeply felt the attention paid by the State Council to the Plan. The National Health and Family Planning Commission led the drafting of the Plan and solicited a dozen of Ministries' opinions for many times. Unlike the previous experience of soliciting opinions among Ministries, the feedback was particularly fast this time and everyone was actively involved. Ministry of Education, Ministry of Agriculture and other Ministries have given very good suggestions, so it can be issued in a year and a half. For the draft submitted by the National Health and Family Planning Commission, the State Council not just approved it, but also made a crucial revision to it. As soon as the Plan was issued, the State Council immediately held a press conference, fully demonstrating that the State

Council has attached great importance to the Plan.

The core content of *National Nutrition Plan* (*2017－2030*) has four parts: general requirements, guiding principles, basic principles, and main goals.

Some highlights are in the basic principles. First, we must adhere to scientific development and give full play to the leading role of science and technology. Second, we must pursue innovation and promote the integration of nutrition and health into industries. It is important to notice that what we emphasize is integration rather than combination. This is in line with the instruction of "driving the development of the food industry" made by Vice Premier LIU Yandong before the drafting work. Therefore, many specific contents in following parts demonstrate the development of the food industry.

Main goals of the *National Nutrition Plan* (*2017–2030*) are divided into two parts, goals by 2020 and goals by 2030, which are in line with some of the health indicators in the *Healthy China 2030 Planning Outline*. For example, pregnant women are deficient in folic acid, and stunting and obesity are both facing the primary and secondary school students. In terms of obesity, the question of "should we set quantitative targets with students as the target population" has been discussed many times in the drafting process. As a result, we all agree that we should seek truth from facts, and only focus on curbing the growth instead of setting quantitative targets. The best result is to make greatest efforts in slowing down the rising trends, rather than set a specific quantitative indicator, as it is estimated that the decline in student obesity rates cannot be achieved by 2020. Therefore, indicator setting and goal setting in the drafting process fully reflect the spirit of seeking truth from facts.

The *National Nutrition Plan* (*2017－2030*) is mainly to tell people how to improve national nutrition and the answer lies in the following seven strategies.

First, improving policy and nutritional law research and strengthen standards. Almost all developed countries and some developing countries have state-level nutritional laws, but China does not have one. So it is hoped to make breakthrough in this regard by implementing the Plan.

Second, improving nutrition capacity building. All the goals are impossible to achieve without enough capacity.

Third, improving the supervision and evaluation of nutrition and food safety.

Fourth, developing the nutrition and health industry with Chinese characteristics. This is the strategy which focuses on food and health industry of nutrition.

Fifth, developing traditional food and nutritional services.

Sixth, enhancing the sharing and use of basic data in nutritional health. National researches have accumulated a large number of data. "How to establish a database to share the data", as one of the proposed strategies, has great guiding significance.

Seventh, popularizing nutrition and health knowledge. This is also a very important strategy. Changing people's behavior holds the key to improve nutrition. People's behavior depends on their own knowledge and cannot be changed without knowledge.

The above seven strategies mainly target the general population, while the following six major actions are targeted at special populations.

First, nutrition and health for the first 1000 days of life. This is the window period. The so-called window period is to improve nutrition within the first 1000 days of life. Of course, it is more than nutrition. But if nutrition is improved in these 1000 days, people will benefit for the whole life. In other words, if nutrition is insufficient in these 1000 days, there will be catch-up growth after birth, which may lead to high prevalence of overweight, obesity, and other chronic diseases, including psychosis, in adulthood. This has been confirmed by scientific researches from home and abroad. So the first 1000 days of life is the first special population.

Second, improving nutrition for students. Students are also a very important special population.

Third, improving nutrition for the elderly. Elderly people have been gradually put on the agenda. Currently, China has not become truly prosperous, but has already entered an aging society. According to the definition of the WHO, China now has more than 200 million elderly people, and this figure will continue to increase by 2030. Problems concerning the elderly are more complex as nutrition, diseases and pension patterns are closely related to each other, and thus improving nutrition for the elderly is very necessary.

Fourth, clinical nutrition. This is also a very important point. For example, if we compare the weight of hospitalized patients on admission and discharge, most patients will lose weight at discharge. In other words, the patient's disease is cured or alleviated, but his or her nutrition is not well improved in the hospital. This is because clinical nutrition has not been given enough attention in the hospital, which relates to various problems such as laws and regulations, public opinions, and whether the hospital directors have paid enough attention to this issue. Compared with developed countries, the status of clinical dietitians in China is much lower, and even much lower than that in Taiwan and Hong Kong. Therefore, great importance has been attached to clinical nutrition improvement. Hospitalized patients must receive a series of targeted measures such as nutrition evaluation and selection to improve their nutrition.

Fifth, improving nutrition for poverty-stricken areas. The emphasis here is on nutrition intervention, as there are many examples of poverty caused by diseases. At the very beginning, experts planned to give top priority to this action and the reason for the State Council to place it to the back was clear, as our country will be fully out of poverty by 2020. Although it is of great importance from a policy point of view, being placed to the back, actually, does not mean that it is not important. In fact, we know very well that if we do not continue to pay attention to the nutrition status of people in these areas after 2020, poverty will happen again.

Sixth, the balance of eating and exercise. Eating is important while physical exercise also should not be ignored.

Besides the above six major actions, the last important part is to strengthen the organization and implementation. There are several points with great significance. For example, local governments at all levels should strengthen the organizational guarantee by including the government's performance appraisal. Conscientiously implementing the *National Nutrition Plan* is not an empty talk. First of all, we must guarantee financial support by increasing investment in *National Nutrition Plan* (*2017 – 2030*). Nutritional issues should rely not just on the government, but more on all kinds of funding channels. In addition, we must also enhance international cooperation, strengthen organization and leadership, and facilitate advocacy and mobilization.

In conclusion, nutrition is a part of modern medicine and is also a part of modern preventive medicine, going hand in hand with health and illness of the people. Implementing the *Healthy China 2030 Planning Outline* and building a moderately prosperous society in all respects cannot be realized without nutrition or more generally, without improved people's nutrition. At present, China has seen the basic needs of over a billion people met, but micronutrient deficiencies still exist. The example just cited is iron deficiency. There are zinc deficiency, iodine deficiency and other problems such as the question of iodized salt and a series of micronutrient deficiencies like calcium, vitamin A and vitamin D. Besides, overweight and obesity are also prominent issues. Therefore, we still have a long way to go.

The *National Nutrition Plan* (*2017–2030*) , issued by the State Council in particular, will play an important role in promoting all-round nutrition work, building a moderately prosperous society in all respects and realizing the dream of healthy China.

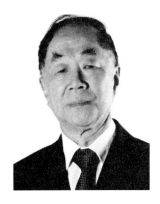

CHEN Junshi is Academician of CAE, Chief Consultant of CFSA, Chairman of the National Expert Committee on Food Safety Risk Assessment, Vice Chairman of the National Food Safety Standards Review Committee, Deputy Director of the Expert Committee of Food Safety Committee of the State Council, Director of health risk assessment and Control of the CPMA, Member of WHO Food Safety Expert Group, Director of China Office of ILSI.

Current Status and Prevention Strategy of Cardiovascular Disease in China

GAO Runlin

National Center of Cardiovascular Diseases, Fuwai Hospital, Chinese Academy of Medical Sciences (CAMS)

Cardiovascular disease has now become the first cause of death among urban and rural residents in China. According to the latest statistics from the National Health and Family Planning Commission of PRC, the mortality of cardiovascular diseases in rural areas accounts for 45% and the urban area accounts for 42%. The death of cardiovascular disease in the country has surpassed that in the city. The burden of cardiovascular disease what our country is facing right now is very heavy.

1   Current status of cardiovascular disease in China

According to estimates from the *Report on Cardiovascular Diseases in China 2014*, the number of China's existing patients with cardiovascular disease is 290 million, among which 270 million people who suffer from hypertension, 7 million people suffer from cerebral stroke, 2.5 million people suffer from myocardial infarction, and 4.5 million suffer from heart failure. And the morbidity and mortality are still on the rise. From 1990 to 2015, cardiovascular mortalities among urban and rural residents in China have been rising; moreover, the mortality is rising faster in rural areas and now has surpassed that in urban areas (see Fig.1).

Cardiovascular diseases include coronary heart disease and cerebrovascular disease. In recent years, the increasing trend in mortality of cerebrovascular disease has slowed down. It has basically trends to flatten in the city; while in the country, it is still rising and even higher than that in the city. According to the age-standardized mortality, it is analyzed that the standardized mortality of cardiovascular diseases is still

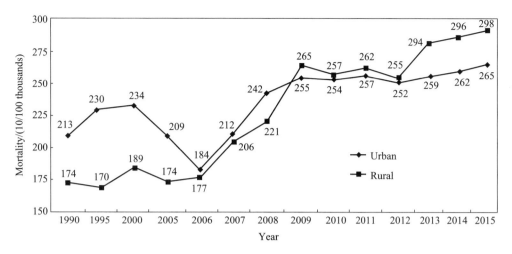

Fig.1 Changes of cardiovascular disease mortality among

urban and rural residents in China from 1990 to 2015

(Quoted from P15 of *Report on Cardiovascular diseases in China 2016*)

increasing, especially the increase of men. Nevertheless, the standardized mortality of cerebral stroke has decreased during 1990 to 2013 (Fig.2), which indicates that our country has achieved initial success in the aspect of preventing and treating cerebral stroke. However, the standardized mortality of coronary heart disease is still on the rise (Fig.3). In the past, it was significantly higher in urban areas than that in rural areas, but they become basically equal now in both areas. In particular, mortalities of acute myocardial infarction in both rural and urban areas have increased significantly, and the mortality in rural areas has increased significantly faster than that in urban areas. Why did this happen? It was mainly due to the changes in people's lifestyle, and the prevalence of risk factors; the prevention and control measures failed to keep up with rapid increase in rural, and the treatment conditions were worse than those in urban areas after catching the disease, which led to the high case fatality rate, with the result that the mortality of myocardial infarction in rural areas is higher than that in urban areas. According to China – PEACE study, the number of myocardial infarction inpatients increased nearly five-fold during the decade of 2001 – 2011 in our country, but the in-hospital mortality of myocardial infarction showed no significant change. The most important treatment to improve the prognosis of myocardial infarction is reperfusion therapy (emergency intervention or thrombolysis). However, in this 10 years, the proportion of reperfusion therapy has remained unchanged and the proportion of emergency intervention has increased, but the proportion of thrombolysis has correspondingly decreased, resulting that the proportion of reperfusion in this 10 years has not changed significantly, which was the main cause of hospital mortality in acute myocardial infarction has not been reduced. According to CAMI registration study, in recent years, proportions of reperfusion therapy in hospitals at all levels have increased, among which proportions in hospitals at provincial-level and above have increased significantly and they were higher than those of city hospitals and county hospitals; meanwhile, the in-hospital mortality of hospitals at provincial-level was significantly lower than that of county hospitals.

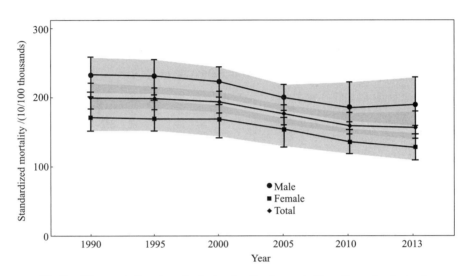

**Fig.2   The variation trend of standardized mortality of cerebral stroke
in China from 1990 to 2013**

(ZHOU M, et al. Lancet. 2016, 387:251-272.)

From 2001 to 2011, the number of cardiovascular inpatients in China has increased five-fold, which significantly increased the economic burden of hospitalization. Compared with developed countries, the cardiovascular control in our country has a long way to go. Let's take the occurrence of cerebral stroke for example. Japan used to be a big country in having cerebral stroke. But, after years of prevention and treatment, the mortality of cerebral stroke has drastically decreased. Nowadays, the mortality of cerebral stroke in China is four times higher than that in Japan and also four times higher than that in the United States, which indicates the task of prevention and control now is very arduous.

According to the "China's Coronary Heart Disease Prediction Model", from 2010 to 2030, if only considering factors in population aging and population increase, the number

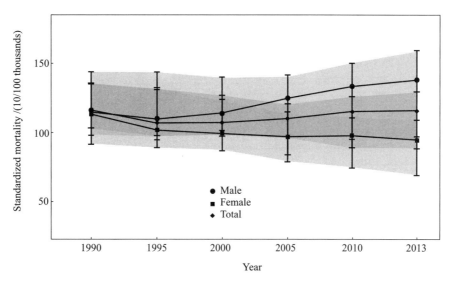

Fig.3 The variation trend of standardized mortality of ischemic heart disease

in China from 1990 to 2013

(ZHOU M,et al. Lancet. 2016,387:251-272.)

of cardiovascular disease events among the population aged 35 to 84 will increase 50%; if considering the factors in hypertension, cholesterol, diabetes, smoking and so on, the number of cardiovascular disease events will additionally increase 23%.

2   China's population aging and risk factors of cardiovascular disease

The cardiovascular disease is mainly caused by aging and risk factors of the cardiovascular disease. Urbanization and aging are inevitable. Since 2005, China has entered an aging society. According to the population aged 65 and above, the elderly population in 2005 was 100 million and by 2017, it was 140 million; while, the population aged over 60 years old has reached 200 million.

Important risk factors for cardiovascular disease include hypertension, high cholesterol, obesity, inadequate intake of fruits and vegetables, smoking, drinking, diabetes, etc., among which the two risk factors of hypertension and high cholesterol are the most important. The contribution rate of cholesterol in developed countries is higher than that of hypertension. For developing countries including China, the contribution rate of hypertension is higher than that of cholesterol, but the contribution rate of cholesterol cannot be ignored as well.

Now, how is it going with the changing situation of risk factors in cardiovascular disease? Based on MUCA's study, more than 80% of cardiovascular diseases in our country (including coronary heart disease and ischemic cerebral stroke) can be attributed to major risk factors, of which 35% are attributed to hypertension, 32% to smoking, 11% to hypercholesterolemia, and 3% to diabetes. The prevalence of hypertension, which is the most important risk factor, is on the rise. In 1959, the prevalence rate in the population aged over 18 was 5.1%; in 1991, it was 12.6%; in 2002, it was 18.8%. For China's major survey project on the prevalence of cardiovascular disease during the 12th Five-Year Plan period, out of a survey sample of 500000 people, the crude prevalence rate of hypertension was 28%, and the weighted rate was 23.2%. The prevalence rate of hypertension in our country is going up all the way, and it increases with age. The prevalence rate is more than 50% in the population aged over 50 and it reaches more than 60% in the population aged over 70. In recent years, prevention and treatment of hypertension have achieved some effect. In accordance with the survey of 2015, the awareness rate of hypertension was 51.5%, treatment rate was 46.1%, and control rate was 16.9%; while in 1991, the awareness rate was only 26%, treatment rate was 12%, and control rate was 3%. Although the level of "three rates" still lags behind that of developed countries, it should be said that the prevention and treatment of hypertension has made some progress under the arrangement of the state with great efforts. Due to the greater relationship between cerebral stroke and hypertension, in recent years, the reduction of standard cerebral stroke mortality in China was at least partly related to the prevention and treatment of hypertension.

Cholesterol is the most important risk factor for coronary heart disease. For the increasing in death of coronary heart disease in Beijing from 1984 to 1999, 77% was due to the increasing of cholesterol. From 1984 to 1999, for Beijing residents, men and women's average cholesterol levels have increased by 24%. The result of lipids test in 2012 showed that people whose LDL cholesterol increasing over 130 mg/dL accounted for 20.4%. If the elevated cholesterol is not strictly controlled, the morbidity of coronary heart disease will increase even further. At present, the prevalence rate of hypercholesterolemia is increasing and the control of hypercholesterolemia is poor. Upon the survey of 17 national community hospitals conducted by PURE's study, the proportion of using statins for secondary prevention of coronary heart disease in China was only 2%, which was much lower than that in Europe and the United States, and merely a little more than that in Africa (1.4%). Of course, it was a sample survey of PURE's study and the sample is not necessarily representative. But it could at least explain that there has been a big gap in our country between using statins for secondary prevention of coronary heart disease and clinical needs. As the relationship between cholesterol increasing and the incidence of coronary heart disease is more closely linked, the fact that standardized mortality of coronary heart disease in China is still rising can be easily understood.

Diabetes is also an important risk factor for cardiovascular disease. In our country, the prevalence rate of diabetes in adults reached 9.7%. In addition, smoking is also an important risk factor for cardiovascular disease in our country. In recent years, under the vigorous smoking-control campaign, the rate of reduction is very limited and the smoking-control work is still not enough. Overweight and obesity are also increasing.

3　Measures on prevention and treatment of cardiovascular disease

3.1　Prevention first, control risk factors

The population aging trend is irresistible, and cannot be changed by us. However, the risk factors can be changed. A series of studies have shown that if the risk factors are under control, 78%–89% incidence of coronary heart disease, 78%–85% death of coronary heart disease, 70%–76% incidence of cerebral stroke, and 65%–73% death of cerebral stroke will be reduced. Therefore, to control cardiovascular and cerebrovascular diseases, we must move forward the front of prevention and treatment, starting with the control of risk factors, and give priority to prevention. Like the old saying, "the superior doctor prevents illness".

There are many successful international examples on reducing the death of cardiovascular diseases by controlling risk factors. From 1968 to 1981, the reduction of cardiovascular mortality in the United States was much more pronounced than that of non-cardiovascular mortality. After World War II, Americans' living standard got improved significantly, including the significant increase in cholesterol intake, which led to an increase in hypertension and explosive growth in cardiovascular deaths. However, because of National Cholesterol Education Program and Hypertension Prevention Program, the mortality of cardiovascular and cerebrovascular diseases has been significantly reduced. Now the mortality of coronary heart disease in the United States has dropped by more than 30% and the cerebral stroke has reduced by nearly 50%. According to the research, for the reduction on mortality of cardiovascular and cerebrovascular diseases in the United States, 65% was attributed to improving risk factors, of which 24% was attributed to lower cholesterol and 20% to the decline of blood pressure of the population. Based on the experience of the United States, effective prevention and control of risk factors, especially controlling hypertension and lowering cholesterol are the most important measures to reduce the death of cardiovascular diseases. Finland was once one of those countries with the highest mortality of cardiovascular disease in the world. Through the research and implementation of North Carolina's Plan, by controlling smoking, changing living habits, and reducing cream intake, Finland has made the mortality of cardiovascular disease in North Carolina and its own country reduce by as much as 80% and 50%, separately. The experience of Finland is well worth learning from.

Our country also has the successful experience of cardiovascular prevention research. Daqing Research started the lifestyle intervention on patients with pre-diabetes in the 1980s. After one year of intervention, the cumulative all-cause mortality after 23-year follow-up was 29% lower than that of the control group. "Shougang" experience showed that by conducting mass prevention and mass treatment to control hypertension could significantly reduce the morbidity and mortality of cerebral stroke.

In 1979, Geoffrey Rose, a famous British epidemiologist, first proposed two strategies to prevent cardiovascular disease: namely the whole population strategy and high-risk population strategy. As Centers for Disease Control and Prevention (CDC) reported, getting the public to acquire knowledge of cardiovascular disease prevention was the most fundamental treatment measure to reduce the morbidity of cardiovascular disease and also the most economical treatment means. In the United States, by changing the lifestyle, the morbidity of hypertension cerebral stroke, diabetes and cancer decreased by 55%, 75%, 50% and 1/3 separately. Moreover, the national life expectancy increased by 10 years.

3.2 Government-leading, "integrating health into all policies"

To prevent and control cardiovascular and cerebrovascular diseases, we must adhere to government-leading. President XI Jinping stressed at the National Health and Fitness Conference: "Put people's health in the position of priority development strategy, and integrate health into all policies". President XI stated that, "We must unswervingly implement the policy of prevention first; adhere to the combination of prevention and control, joint prevention and control, mass prevention and control; and make great efforts to provide health and wellness services for the people in their whole life cycles." President Xi's important instructions also pointed out the direction for the prevention and treatment of cardiovascular diseases. For cardiovascular disease, as the most common chronic disease, in order to effectively control the occurrence of it, the prevention and control work must be led by the government; prevention and treatment should be moved forward; prevention should be put first.

3.3　Strengthen the construction of hierarchical diagnosis and treatment system

In order to effectively prevent and control cardiovascular disease, it is very important to strengthen the construction of hierarchical diagnosis and treatment system. There are about 290 million people suffering from cardiovascular disease and at least 270 million of them have hypertension. As mentioned earlier, hypertension is the most important risk factor cardiovascular disease. If 50% of hypertensive patients visit tertiary hospitals, then each hospital will have to receive 320 hypertensive patients daily. As a result, the hospital will be overwhelmed and the doctor will have no time to fully communicate with patients, let alone doing follow-up. Conducting hierarchical diagnosis and treatment can effectively solve this problem. Therefore, we should emphasize proceeding the first visit at the grassroots level, and strength the cooperation between superior and junior hospitals. For people living in the community, if they have hypertension, most of them can be early diagnosed by the community medical institution; patients with general hypertension can be given treatment; the institution will do followed-up visits for hypertensive patients and observe their treatment effects. If the patient's blood pressure is not well controlled, he/she can be transferred to the secondary hospital; the secondary hospital can adjust the patient's drugs according to the guideline. If the patient's condition is difficult to deal with for the secondary hospital, he/she can be transferred to the tertiary hospital and specialized hospital for further examination and adjusting the treatment; if necessary, further tests should be conducted to rule out secondary hypertension. After the patient's blood pressure is stable, he/she can be transferred back to the secondary hospital or community medical institution, and given long-term follow-up visits as to observe treatment effects. In this way, we can build an effective system of prevention and control of hypertension. The community should organize health education activities to popularize the knowledge about preventing hypertension, and give residents regular inspections so as to early detect hypertensive patients and improve the rates of hypertensive awareness and treatment. Thereby the morbidity and mortality of cerebral stroke and coronary heart disease can effectively reduce.

Hypertension is a chronic disease and its grading diagnosis and treatment is from the bottom to the top; while for acute myocardial infarction, an acute disease with high mortality, its grading diagnosis and treatment should be from the top to the bottom. If there is a patient with acute chest pain and suspected myocardial infarction, we should immediately call an ambulance, begin to contact the hospital, and then send him/she to the hospital with emergency invention (PCI) condition for emergency PCI through the green channel ASAP. If the patient is sent to a hospital without PCI condition, he/she should be performed thrombolytic therapy ASAP, then transferred to a superior hospital for coronary angiography, and conducted PCI if necessary. After the patient is stable, he/she can be transferred to the secondary hospital for rehabilitation. In this way, the proportion of reperfusion therapy can be increased, the time from the first medical exposure to reperfusion can be shortened, and the mortality of acute myocardial infarction can be reduced.

3.4 Implement standardized management of chronic diseases

Another problem is to regulate the management of chronic disease, and the standard must be implemented. First, we should formulate standards, guidelines, clinical pathways for chronic disease management. The health managements of hypertension and diabetes have been listed in national financial appropriation, which has covered contents of free national basic public health service projects (for all residents). As a recent published survey showed, out of 3362 primary care units, 8.1% of hospitals had no antihypertensive at all and only 33.8% of the units had four types of antihypertensive confirmed to be effective by evidence-based medicine. If there is no medicine, how can we conduct the control of hypertension? Therefore, the implementation of policy is very important.

3.5 Promote the transformation from "medical insurance" to "health insurance"

The last point is about medical insurance problem. We should promote the transition from medical insurance to health insurance. Right now, our medical insurance is mainly used to protect the people who need treatment and it cost huge. The current standardized mortality of coronary heart disease is on the rise, and these terminally ill patients are going to spend a lot of medical insurance funds. If we control hypercholesterolemia from the upstream, the morbidity of coronary heart disease can be reduced by 20%. Hypercholesterolemia has no symptoms, and if the patient doesn't take tests, he/she will not notice it. Thus, the awareness rate of this disease is very low. Usually even the patient knowing have it, he/she may not get suitable treatment. If the important risk factor—high cholesterol cannot be controlled, how can coronary heart disease be controlled? So we suggest managing the "three high" together. Now that hypertension and diabetes have been included in basic health service projects, we recommend including hypercholesterolemia as well. In this way, risk factors can be more effectively controlled and cardiovascular mortality will be reduced. This means that the department of health should change the concept and perform the transition from medical security to health security.

3.6 Promote the role of "Internet+"

In addition, we use Internet technology to do health education for patients and the public, training of primary doctors, tele-consultation platform, and medical guidance through hospital union. "Internet+" will play an important role.

4 Conclusions

Cardiovascular disease is the first cause of death among urban and rural residents in China, and the mortality is still on the rise. The rise of cardiovascular mortality is mainly due to the aging of the population and the prevalence of risk factors; hypertension, hypercholesterolemia, diabetes, smoking, overweight-obesity and other factors are the most important risk factors. The key to prevent and treat cardiovascular disease is to prevent and control risk factors, which should be done as follows: adhere to government-leading, prevent first, implement standard management of prevention and treatment, establish hierarchical diagnosis and treatment system, promote the transformation from "medical insurance" to "health insurance" and give full play to the role of "Internet+". The inflection point in the reduction of cardiovascular mortality in China will come soon.

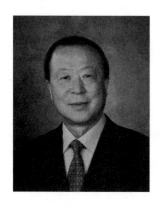

GAO Runlin is a cardiovascular expert. He graduated from Beijing Medical University in 1965 and obtained a master's degree from Peking Union Medical College in 1981. He was the Director of Institute of Cardiovascular Disease and Fuwai Cardiovascular Hospital (Chinese Academy of Medical Sciences) , and also the Chief of Cardiology Department; he is Chairman of Expert Committee of National Center of Cardiovascular Diseases, Chief Expert of Cardiology Department of Fuwai Hospital, researcher, doctoral supervisor. In 1999, he was elected as Academician of Chinese Academy of Engineering.

GAO has been working in the clinical front line over a long period of time; he has been engaged in clinic, scientific research and crowd prevention and control work of cardiovascular disease; and he is one of the pioneers of interventional cardiology in China. He has made many contributions, like establishing and developing interventional cardiology; popularizing, promoting, standardizing and producing domestic equipment of coronary heart disease interventional therapy. As a major researcher, he has completed the science and technology supporting project of 12th Five-Year Plan—the morbidity survey and key technology research of China's major cardiovascular disease.

Healthy China—Early Treatment Strategy for Respiratory Diseases

ZHONG Nanshan

National Clinical Research Center for Respiratory Disease, Guangzhou Medical University

Today, respiratory diseases are seriously threatening the health of the Chinese people. In China, main factors affecting respiratory system include severe air pollution, smoking and frequent major acute respiratory diseases. Chronic diseases account for 87% of China's total deaths and chronic respiratory diseases account for 11%[1], seriously threatening the health of the Chinese people. Prevention and control of respiratory diseases is a major demand for the Healthy China strategy. China's clinical prevention and treatment strategy should develop from the "4P" mode, namely Predictive, Preventive, Personalized and Participatory, to the "5P" mode by adding Presymptomatic.

Smoking is a risk factor for respiratory diseases. Tobacco consumption was initially higher in California than in other states, but it declined as tobacco control policy went into effect. Thanks to 40 years of carrying out this policy, there has been a significant drop of tobacco consumption in California compared to other states[2]. After nearly 50 years of development from 1960 to 2007, smoking rate of China maintains at a high level and did not show significant decline as presented by the US, the UK and Japan, as shown in Fig.1.

In addition to smoking, air pollution is also an important risk factor that cannot be ignored in the high incidence of respiratory diseases in China. In this regard, a study of the association between air pollution and chronic obstructive pulmonary disease (COPD) was conducted during the period of 2012 – 2015 by including registered population aged 20 in two streets or villages which had been randomly selected from

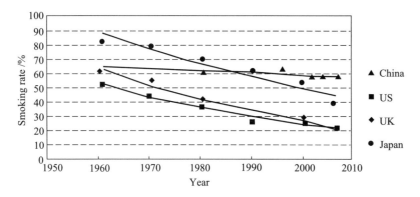

Fig.1 Smoking rate of males in some countries

four cities respectively in Guangdong Province (Guangzhou and Zhanjiang represent urban area, and Shaoguan and Heyuan represent rural area). The study showed that the prevalence of COPD is significantly correlated with PM concentration[3]. As PM2.5 concentration rises from 35 mg/m^3 to 75 mg/m^3, the risk of COPD increases by 2.416 times; as PM10 concentration rises from 50 mg/m^3 to 150 mg/m^3, the risk of COPD increases by 2.442 times. This means that for each 10 mg/m^3 increase in PM2.5, FEV1 decreases by 25 mL. Therefore, air pollution poses a great threat to the respiratory system.

Diagnosis and treatment of lung cancer should improve the diagnosis rate of early lung cancer to reduce the overall mortality of lung cancer so as to achieve early detection and early intervention. The 5-year survival rate gets lower as the stage of lung cancer becomes later[4]. Therefore, early screening of lung cancer is of great significance to early prevention and early treatment. Recently, with the support of the People's Government of Guangzhou Municipality, Health and Family Planning Commission of Guangzhou Municipality and Bureau of Civil Affairs of Guangzhou Municipality, headed by the First Affiliated Hospital of Guangzhou Medical University and the National Clinical Research Center for Respiratory Diseases, a free lung cancer screening project was launched for low-income people and residents living in Yuexiu District, Guzhangzhou Municipality with the help of the community network, providing free low-cost spiral CT and tumor markers tests for eligible residents. This project aimed at increasing the diagnosis rate of early lung cancer so as to reduce the overall mortality rate of lung cancer. In addition to early screening, the thoracic surgery team of the Guangzhou Institute of Respiratory Disease also analyzed clinical features associated with relapse concerning the clinical issues of postoperative recurrence of lung cancer at early stages, and identified relevant genes of tumor based on the nomogram of clinical factors. It developed a multi-gene expression-based prediction model through L2 COX and published two survival prediction models globally[5-6]. To some extent, this can be seen as a clinical prediction approach to improve the prognosis of lung cancer.

In 2015, about 3.2 million people died of COPD worldwide, an increase of 11.6%[7] over 1990. Long-term maintenance treatment strategy of COPD should focus on early lesions, because patients with early stages of COPD account for the highest proportion (i.e. GOLD Stages I–II). Patients with GOLD Stages I–II account for 76%[8] of all COPD patients in the US and for almost 70.7%[9] in China. *GOLD 2006* abolished the GOLD Stage 0, because there was insufficient evidence to support that GOLD Stage 0 patients would progress to GOLD Stage I patients[10]. But according to the latest research, GOLD Stage 0 is close to GOLD Stage I concerning quality of life and capacity of physical activity[11], and more than 50% of people with GOLD Stage 0 have respiratory-related impairments. By OCT (optical coherence tomography technology to detect small airway lesions), it can be found that quite a number of heavy smokers, though with normal lung function, have a changed small airway structure[12], which can be seen as evidence for the GOLD Stage 0.

COPD patients generally develop symptoms only when FEV1 declines significantly (FEV1 ⩽ 50%)[13]. Compared with healthy people, all patients with different GOLD Stages may show yearly rate of decline in peak FEV1 and patients with GOLD Stages I–II may show more obvious decline[14 16] which means that lung function of early stages of COPD decreases faster. Therefore, early stages of COPD have the following features: small airways lesion is the most prominent feature with slight symptoms which are often ignored; exercise tolerance has declined; and the rate of decline in FEV1 is the fastest.

Most important strategies of COPD treatment include early detection and early treatment. *GOLD 2018* points out that COPD is a common, preventable and treatable disease that is characterized by persistent respiratory symptoms and airflow limitation that is due to airway and/or alveolar abnormalities usually caused by significant exposure to noxious particles or gases. According to the definition, COPD should be considered in any patient who has dyspnea, chronic cough or sputum production, and/ or a history of exposure to risk factors for the disease. Spirometry is required to make the diagnosis (the presence of a post-bronchodilator FEV1/FVC <0.70). The focus of the report is on the diagnosis after symptoms appear. China has seen severe under-diagnosis and under-treatment of COPD. Only 35.1% of all patients diagnosed as COPD in the study were previously diagnosed as COPD, which indicates under-diagnosis of COPD; even for Stage II patients with milder disease, 64.7% of whom have at least one respiratory symptom while mostly have not received treatment, which indicates under-treatment of COPD[9].

Guangzhou Institute of Respiratory Disease of the First Affiliated Hospital of Guangzhou Medical University conducted a randomized, double-blind, parallel-group, multi-center trial. Patients with GOLD Stages I–II (symptom-free or with very slight symptoms) were selected through the primary screening of COPD and were randomly assigned to receive either tiotropium bromide or matching placebo for 2 years. The difference of trough FEV1 at 24 months from baseline is the primary outcome measure of this study. Study results show that tiotropium bromide continues to significantly improve FEV1 and FVC in patients compared with placebo, and the yearly rate of decline in peak FEV1 is lower in the tiotropium group than in the placebo group. Compared with placebo, tiotropium bromide significantly reduces the risk of first COPD exacerbation, prolonged the time to first COPD exacerbation, and decreases rates of exacerbation/hospitalization so as to continuously improve patients' quality of life[17]. Tie–COPD is the first prospective study of early intervention with tiotropium bromide in patients with COPD (GOLD Stages I–II, symptom-free or with very slight symptoms). Tiotropium bromide can continuously and significantly improve lung function and slow the yearly rate of decline in peak FEV1 (including CAT <10, i.e., patients with no obvious symptoms). It can also improve the quality of life and reduce the number of acute exacerbations. Medical intervention in patients with early stages of COPD can bring clinical benefits, providing more evidence for early prevention and early treatment of diseases and reducing the burden of patients and the society. Follow-up shows that there is no difference in FEV1 after 12 months of discontinuation of tiotropium bromide between the two groups, indicating that even patients with early stages of COPD require continuous intervention. The recent GOLD Report recommends case-finding in patients with symptoms, but not in asymptomatic population. The US Preventive Services Task Force (USPSTF) also does not recommend screening for COPD in asymptomatic adults[18]. I do not share this opinion. The Tie – COPD trial recommends that people (even asymptomatic) exposed to risk factors (e. g., smoking, cooking with biofuels, and exposure to severe air pollution) for a long time should conduct screening spirometry. It also found that patients with early stages of COPD require continuous treatment. This is similar to early intervention strategy of hypertension and diabetes, and is also the new strategy of early intervention in COPD diagnosis and treatment.

At the National Health and Fitness Conference in 2016, President XI Jinping stated the guidelines for promoting health and fitness services: "focus on lower-level medical institutions, strive to reform and make innovations in the medical sector, prioritize disease prevention, lay equal emphasis on Western medicine and TCM, incorporate health promotion in all policies, and involve all citizens in promoting public health and thereby bring health benefits to all." If one does not pay attention to early prevention and early treatment, and receives treatment or even rescue only after symptoms appear, medical costs will definitely rise; on the contrary, if one pays much attention to early prevention and early treatment, and reduce the chance of receiving treatment or rescue after symptoms appear, medical costs will surely decline. Therefore, China's clinical prevention and treatment strategy should be developed towards early prevention and early intervention.

References

[1] WHO. Noncommunicable diseases: country profiles 2014. 2014.

[2] PIERCE J P, MESSER K, WHITE M M, et al. Forty years of faster decline in cigarette smoking in California explains current lower lung cancer rates. Cancer Epidemiology, Biomarkers & Prevention,2010,19:2801-2810.

[3] LIU S, ZHOU Y, LIU S, et al. Association between exposure to ambient particulate matter and chronic obstructive pulmonary disease: results from a cross-sectional study in China. Thorax,2017,72:788-795.

[4] DETTERBECK F C, BOFFA D J, TANOUE LT. The new lung cancer staging system. Chest,2009,136:260-271.

[5] LIANG W, ZHANG L, JIANG G, et al. Development and validation of a nomogram for predicting survival in patients with resected non-small-cell lung cancer. Journal of Clinical Oncology,2015,33:861-869.

[6] KRATZ J R, HE J, VAN DEN EEDEN S K, et al. A practical molecular assay to predict survival in resected non-squamous, non-small-cell lung cancer: development and international validation studies. Lancet, 2012, 379:823-832.

[7] SORIANO J B, ABAJOBIR A A, ABATE K H, et al. Global, regional, and national deaths, prevalence, disability-adjusted life years, and years lived with disability for chronic obstructive pulmonary disease and asthma, 1990-2015: a systematic analysis for the Global Burden of Disease Study 2015. Lancet Respiratory Medicine,2017,5:691-706.

[8] MAPEL D W, DALAL A A, BLANCHETTE C M, et al. Severity of COPD at initial spirometry-confirmed diagnosis: data from medical charts and administrative claims. International Journal of Chronic Obstructive Pulmonary Disease,2011,6:573-581.

[9] ZHONG N, WANG C, YAO W, et al. Prevalence of chronic obstructive pulmonary disease in China: a large, population-based survey. American Journal of Respiratory and Critical Care Medicine,2007,176:753-760.

[10] VESTBO J, LANGE P. Can GOLD Stage 0 provide information of prognostic value in chronic obstructive pulmonary disease. American Journal of Respiratory and Critical Care Medicine,2002,166:329-332.

[11] REGAN E A, LYNCH D A, CURRAN-EVERETT D, et al. Clinical and radiologic disease in smokers with normal spirometry. JAMA Internal Medicine,2015,175:1539-1549.

[12] DING M, CHEN Y, GUAN W J, et al. Measuring airway remodeling in patients with different COPD staging using endobronchial optical coherence tomography. Chest,2016,150:1281-1290.

[13] SUTHERLAND E R, CHERNIACK R M. Management of chronic obstructive pulmonary disease. The New England Journal of Medicine,2004,350:2689-2697.

[14] WELTE T, VOGELMEIER C, PAPI A. COPD: early diagnosis and treatment to slow disease progression. International Journal of Clinical Practice,2015,69:336-349.

[15] TANTUCCI C, MODINA D. Lung function decline in COPD. International Journal of Chronic Obstructive Pulmonary Disease,2012,7:95-99.

[16] PITTA F, TROOSTERS T, SPRUIT M A, et al. Characteristics of physical activities in daily life in chronic obstructive pulmonary disease. American Journal of Respiratory and Critical Care Medicine,2005,171:972-977.

[17] ZHOU Y, ZHONG N S, LI X, et al. Tiotropium in early-stage chronic obstructive pulmonary disease. The New England Journal of Medicine,2017,377:923-935.

[18] FORCE USPST, SIU A L, BIBBINS-DOMINGO K, et al. Screening for chronic obstructive pulmonary disease: US preventive services task force recommendation statement. JAMA,2016,315:1372-1377.

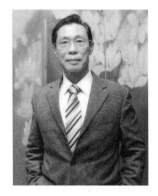

Zhong Nanshan is Academician of Chinese Academy of Engineering, Director of the National Center for Clinical Research in Respiratory Diseases, professor and doctoral tutor of Respiratory Medicine, Guangzhou Medical University, Chief Scientist of "973" project, President and Consultant of Chinese Medical Association, Honorary Professor of University of Edinburgh, Doctor of Science University of Birmingham, a senior member of the Royal Society of Medicine (Edinburgh, London), the first Hong Kong Centennial Distinguished Scholar.

Health in All Policies—Why and How

Evelyne de Leeuw

Centre for Health Equity Training, Research and Evaluation

A popular saying claims that only two things in life are certain: death and taxes. This is a good metaphor for the current state of play in the global perspectives on health policy and health promotion. Although on average the world's people are enjoying increased life expectancy, there are two problems with living longer. The first is that the years added to life are not necessarily all good quality years. In most societies around the world, we see a concentration of ill health (and notably an accumulation of chronic conditions of the so-called non-communicable diseases) in the last quarter of the life span. For most people now looking forward to live to beyond 80 years of age, sixteen of these will be spent in ill health. But there is another factor at play which makes this problem even more poignant. There are significant inequities in health, not just in life expectancy (a very crude measure of population health) but also-and more importantly-inequities in quality of life and years of life lived in good health. For each of these there is what is called a "social gradient"[1]—those with better social position, better work, better income, better education, better social support systems, are also better off in health. They live longer, and in the years that they live longer, they are also healthier.

This has very little to do with actual individual lifestyle choices, contrary to what most preventative health policies around the world want us to believe. There is very little individual discretionary potential in choosing social position, better work, higher incomes, the best possible education, and good quality housing, legal support, security systems, etc. All of these contributors to better health (also known as the social, political and commercial determinants of health) depend on collective choice, on how our collective systems (be they called the State, a Mutuality Christian community, or Ummah Muslim structure) (re)distribute their resources. This is, indeed, about taxes. And not all taxes are equal. In some countries taxes and levies on unhealthy products (e.g., tobacco, alcohol, or sugary drinks) are significant, and feed back into financing health promotion systems. This happens at the state level in Australia, and at the local level in Korea. In other countries general taxes finance universal health care systems and other welfare constellations (e.g., parental leave) whereas in other countries such provisions are absent and are left to individuals to arrange. Such distributive and redistributive policies are not necessarily driven by the existing evidence base to support and create healthy and thriving populations.

We know, for instance, that significant public health interventions are the best social investment imaginable. Traditionally, such investments include vaccination programmes and seatbelt requirements. For each monetary unit investment they yield many more in return. But it is in particular outside the traditional health care realm that great health investments can be identified. A monetary unit invested in girls' literacy programmes yields vastly more health than the same unit invested in medical care.

Back to colloquialisms and popular proverbs. Although death and taxes are certain, we all similarly embrace sayings like "an apple a day keeps the doctor away". The evidence, however, clearly indicates that governments do not see a prominent role for themselves in the implementation of this wisdom. In a study by the Dutch national Institute of Public Health and the Environment authors highlighted that a fraction of the public sector health budget is spent on prevention, and only a fraction of that spent on health promotion. Consequently, nations around the world spend extraordinary amounts on the disease sector—spending money on fixing problems expensively that could have been avoided in the first place, or extending lives at great cost but not with great returns in terms of quality of life. In a way, we could say that state health care budgets are wasteful, and do not deliver health. This is most notable in the case of the United States of America which has arguably the most expensive health care system in the world, but also one of the most underperforming and inequitable health care systems in the world (Fig.1).

1 What creates health (equity)?

If governments were to take their task seriously to protect and improve the health of their people—and do this equitably for all so no group in society falls behind—it is important to have an understanding of what it is that creates health. This is a quite

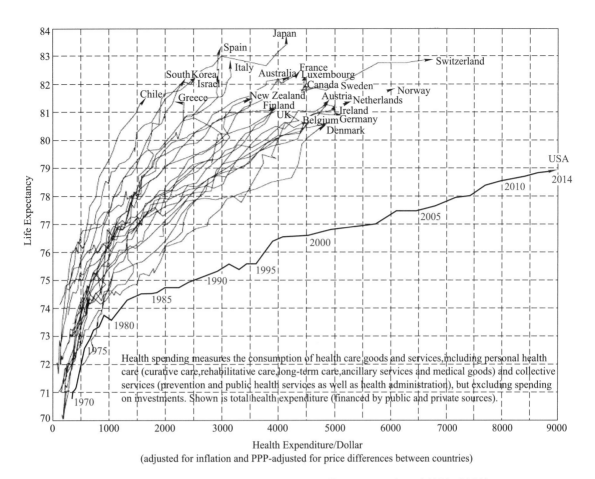

Fig.1 Life expectancy vs. health expenditure over time（1970-2014）

different question from "what creates disease"—mostly addressed in the biomedical sciences. The latter is more or less easily answered in a pathological Cartesian frame of mind, looking at a range of pathogens (e. g., viruses, toxins, etc.). But to ask what creates and sustains "health" for populations is an entirely different question.

One of the first to consider this was Professor Henrik Blum in the late 1960s and early 1970s [2]—who incidentally worked with Hubert Laframboise[3] of Health Canada's Long Range Health Planning Branch—the man that was instrumental in the development and publication of the now famous 1974 government paper "A New Perspective on the Health of Canadians". Also known as "The Lalonde Report" (after the Minister who advocated for it) this document was the first to explicitly acknowledge that in the "health field" human biology, lifestyle, health care and environment work together to create health. The more fine-grained view (Fig.2) obviously shows that there is much more detail to such an idea than just four "fields"—and it does not really do justice to the dynamics between determinants of health.

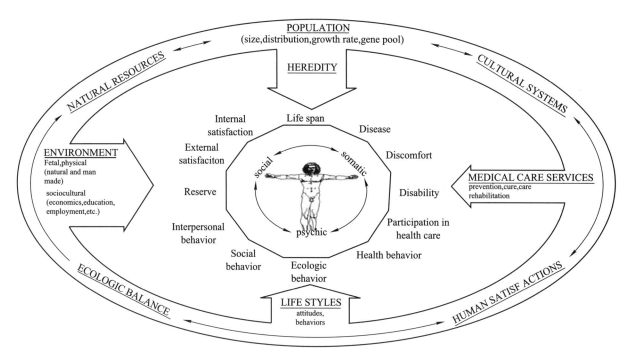

Fig.2　Henrik Blum's version of the Health Field Concept[2]

This challenge was much later taken up by another Canadian team[4] that tried to explain the social gradient in health. The endeavoured to map the pathways that lead to differential health outcomes between populations (Fig.3). Although there are physiological routes, too (and they may be amenable to lifestyle change and even pharmaceutical intervention), the key finding is that social and environmental systems play very important roles in shaping health opportunities and positive health [5]. In turn this means that there is a role for social systems like (local, regional and national) governments but also private workplaces to set standards and policies that create and sustain health.

This is of course not a new insight. Dahlgren and Whitehead[6], based on work commissioned by the World Health Organization in the 1980s, published their widely popular "rainbow" social model of health and health equity (Fig.4). But even before that, First Nations communities around the world knew that harmony, balance and socio-ecological systems are essential for building and maintaining health (Fig.5).

2　We don't want more problems but more solutions

For as long as the social determinants argument has been made, academics and policy actors (not to speak about community activists) have been concerned about

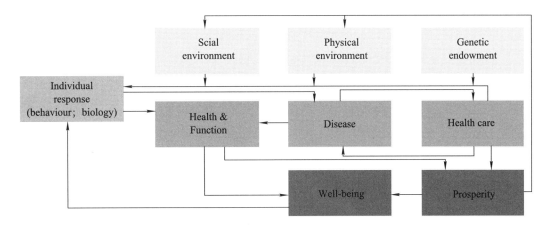

Fig.3　From "What Makes Some People Healthy and Others Not" [4]

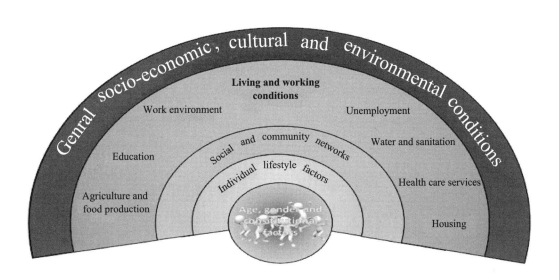

Fig.4　Margaret Whitehead's and Göran Dahlgren's popular Rainbow Model
of determinants of health: the "layers of influence"

addressing this problem which was found to be socially and morally unjust [7]. The World Health Organization and member states like Finland, Sweden, Denmark, and the Netherlands all studied the social determinants of health and health inequalities for policy development reasons [8]. Generally, like the United States, the United Kingdom, and Australia, they agreed that this complex problem required complex solutions. For example, the British government's consultation paper *Tackling Health Inequalities in England* notes: "The Acheson Report examined the determinants of health as 'layers of influence' ⋯ Tackling health inequalities will require us to address all of these 'layers of influence'", and the 2002 Wales health policy recognizes that "to reduce health

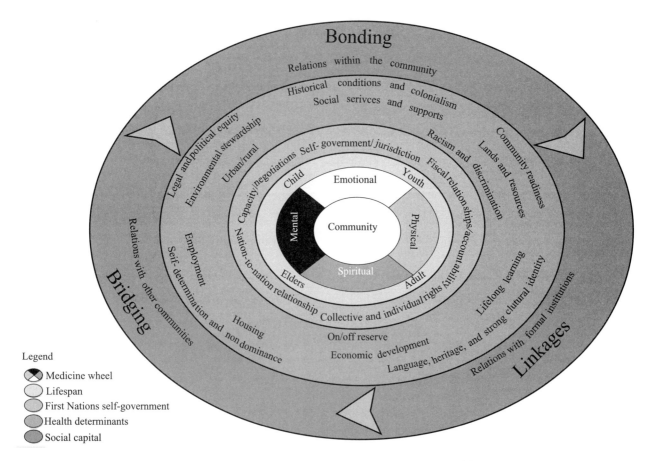

Fig.5　A First Nations determinants of health map [8]

inequalities a multi-faceted strategy is required ⋯ to tackle the economic and environmental determinants of health" [8].

It seems, however, that very few countries (or lower level governments) have actually delivered on such insights. Comprehensive government programmes that specifically and thoughtfully analyse and identify levers for better health in the different multi-dimensional multi-faceted layers of causation are still rare—although the academic literature on social determinants of health and health equity is exploding (Fig.6).

Governments are clearly struggling with the idea that "layers of influence" extend to all disciplinary and government domains, and that the development and sustainability of equitable population health must involve much more than the health care sector alone.

An early identification in terms of policy solutions cam from the Ottawa Charter for Health Promotion in 1986, which adopted a vision to "Build Healthy Public Policy" (a term coined simultaneously by Nancy Milio[9] and Trevor Hancock[10]. In serendipity they came up with the term "Healthy Public Policy" in the mid-1980s[11]. Milio went on to

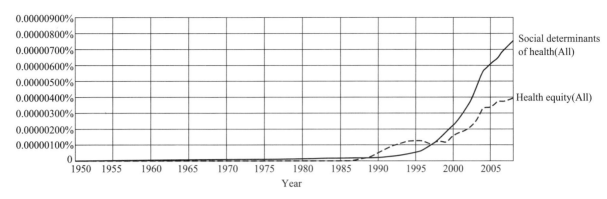

Fig.6 Frequency of the occurrence of the phrases "social determinants of health" and "health equity" in the total corpus of English language books indexed by Google

author the seminal book "Promoting Health Through Public Policy" which had a major impact on the development of the Ottawa Charter for Health Promotion[12]. In this call for a new public health, the Charter recognised that promoting health required enabling, mediating and promoting of a reorientation of health services, development of supportive environments for health, and community action as well as personal skills. To support and reinforce these health promotion strategies, the Charter identified that Healthy Public Policies were required—that is, policies at every level of government that take positive and/or adverse effects on health explicitly into account[13]. The Health Promotion Glossary [14] describes Healthy Public Policy as "…characterized by an explicit concern for health and equity in all areas of policy, and by an accountability for health impact. The main aim of healthy public policy is to create a supportive environment to enable people to lead healthy lives. Such a policy makes healthy choices possible or easier for citizens. It makes social and physical environments health enhancing."

Fafard believes that such a perspective on "a wide range of policies and program interventions that seek to make real change in the wide range of health determinants both at the national and international level" is "perplexing as it leads to a definition that encompasses most of what governments do (and beyond)." [15] Marmor and Boyum [16] make the point even more succinctly: "It is naive to assume that identifying a cause of ill health—like poverty—does much in itself to mobilize action against economic want."

Perhaps the Ottawa Charter, and Milio's identification of the full spectrum of government sectors potentially impacting on health, reflected an idealistic Zeitgeist in which there was a strong belief and confidence in the makeability of society and the power of rational approaches to evidence-based policy. But the lasting legacy of the

Ottawa Charter also shows that the visionary perspective has considerable appeal [17]. Regardless, there is very little empirical evidence on the success or failure of the development and impact of Healthy Public Policy with the exception of initiatives at the local level [18]. Most scholarly authorship on Healthy Public Policy remains abstract and rhetorical [19] and devoid of foundation in policy studies and political science [20].

The recognition of the fact that health determinants lie outside the sphere of the health sector has led to repeated calls for intersectoral action, in earnest starting with the adoption of the Alma Ata Declaration of Primary Health Care, but decreasing after the adoption of the Ottawa Charter for Health Promotion and the regression of a more comprehensive (horizontal) view of primary health care to efforts to frame the concept as being applicable to specific disease management programmes.

Intersectoral health, as strongly advocated by the World Health Organization, and argued consistently over several decades now, is needed to improve the health of populations. A 1986 report [21] provides insights how other sectors contribute to health and development. The report was a co-production between WHO and the Office of the Director-General for Development and International Economic Cooperation, United Nations; the United Nations Environment Programme (UNEP); the United Nations Centre for Human Settlements (Habitat) and the International Year of Shelter for the Homeless (IYSH); the Food and Agriculture Organization of the United Nations (FAO); and the United Nations Educational, Scientific and Cultural Organization (UNESCO). It appears no significant progress has been made, as the statement on the Eight Global Conference on Health Promotion in Helsinki in 2013 includes a similar array of partners, e.g., OECD, the United Nations Development Programme, the International Organization for Migration, etc., with similar recommendations. To quote the 1986 report: "… efforts point to the potential resources that are available for health promotion through intersectoral action. But it cannot be said that they have as yet led to a comprehensive intersectoral approach that would enable the health sector to collaborate with other sectors to shape and influence their health-related components towards a positive outcome in health."

In the 30 years since this first significant effort to document and change the involvement of other sectors in health there has also been a substantive growth in rhetoric that addresses the problem. From different disciplines and fields there have been calls to establish-beyond the (multi) (inter) (cross) sectoral jargon-Joined-Up

Government (JUG), Whole-of-Government (WOG), and integrated governance [22] and other comprehensive ideas to align distinct and separate views, disciplines, public sectors and industry delineations toward health.

3　Health in All Policies—beyond the rhetoric?

Although Milio has demonstrated that virtually every walk of life, public policy and civil society impacts on individual and population health the most significant sectors that have been singled out persistently are:

- education;
- housing and urban planning;
- transport and mobility;
- social protection and welfare support systems;
- energy and sustainable development [23].

Around the world governments at all levels have experimented with integrated health policies[24]. Some of these actually inspired the pronouncements of the Ottawa Charter, e.g., the Norwegian Farm – Food – Nutrition policy, the Chinese "barefoot doctors" programme, and women's health initiatives in the Americas. Two initiatives, on opposite ends of the world started the developmental process of what now is called Health in All Policies (HiAP). During the Presidency of Finland of the European Union the country, building on its effective experience in the long-running North Karelia project (labelled a "horizontal health policy"), urged other members of the Union to engage in

"…a horizontal, complementary policy-related strategy contributing to improved population health. The core of HiAP is to examine determinants of health that can be altered to improve health but are mainly controlled by the policies of sectors other than health."

Almost simultaneously, the government of the state of South Australia, guided by its "Thinker in Residece" Professor Ilona Kickbusch, identified opportunities for a broad policy programme to invest in the health of its people:

"Health in All Policies aims to improve the health of the population through increasing the positive impacts of policy initiatives across all sectors of government and at the same time contributing to the achievement of other sectors' core goals."

These two developments provided impetus for the organization of the Eight Global Conference on Health Promotion (Helsinki, June 2013) where a statement and framework were adopted that expressed HiAP as follows:

"Health in All Policies is an approach to public policies across sectors that systematically takes into account the health implications of decisions, seeks synergies, and avoids harmful health impacts in order to improve population health and health equity. It improves accountability of policymakers for health impacts at all levels of policy-making. It includes an emphasis on the consequences of public policies on health systems, determinants of health and well-being."

In different countries and jurisdictions the emphases of the different dimensions of HiAP vary. Consistently, values associated with the concept centre around the importance of collaboration between sectors of public policy-making in good partnership. Other aspects where less coherence exist between the different jurisdictions include health equity, the attainment of synergy, HiAP leading to or driven by accountability, the character of innovation, ways of integration and the very nature of policy, e.g. [25]:

"Health in All Policies is a collaborative approach that integrates and articulates health considerations into policy making across sectors, and at all levels, to improve the health of all communities and people."—US Association of State and Territorial Health Officers (ASTHO).

"Health in All Policies is a collaborative approach to improving the health of all people by incorporating health considerations into decision-making across sectors and policy areas." — California Health in All Policies Task Force.

"Health in All Policies is the policy practice of including, integrating or internalizing health in other policies that shape or influence the [Social Determinants of Health (SDoH)] …Health in All Policies is a policy practice adopted by leaders and policy makers to integrate consideration of health, well-being and equity during the development, implementation and evaluation of policies."—European Observatory on Health Systems and Policies.

"Health in All Policies is an innovative, systems change approach to the processes through which policies are created and implemented."—National Association of County and City Health Officials (NACCHO).

As a consequence of the adoption, in 2014, of World Health Assembly Resolution 67.12 ("Contributing to social and economic development: sustainable action across sectors to improve health and health equity") a global process of consultation and deliberation has been initiated that should lead to further consistency and priority setting. HiAP as a global and local ("glocal") culmination of development.

As stated above, HiAP is firmly grounded in several decades of evolution of thinking around health development and health promotion, increased sophistication in discerning the causes (of the causes) of health and disease, a further prominence of considerations around sustainability and resilience for human development, and a firmer position of health (in) equ(al) ity issues on local, national and global agendas as well as across diverse populations, including gender and Indigenous populations. The discussions around these issues often take a rights-based and value-driven orientation as affirmed consistently by UN and WHO resolutions at the global and regional level.

Clearly, as has been argued for instance in the Ottawa Charter for Health Promotion—and in fact the Constitution of WHO—these include fundamental prerequisites to health (peace, shelter, education, food, income, a stable eco-system, sustainable resources, social justice, and equity) that interconnect and pervade a broader development agenda.

The five sectors that kicked off this section have been explored and mapped in-depth as having significant potential to impact on people's health in economically feasible and advantageous ways. It should be observed, though, that economic evaluations of intersectoral approaches to social determinants of health generally fail to address distributional (equity) effects across the existing social gradients; economic arguments on health challenges seem to be a policy-critical frame or pitch for successful engagement in horizontal public policy efforts.

The question for the public health community is how to engage with these other sectors for mutual health and development benefit. A WHO report [26] suggests there are three types of "interventions" at the interface of sectoral interests (Fig. 7).

The Venn diagram in Fig. 7 suggests the need to develop a more bespoke and differentiated view of what "Health in All Policies" are, can and should be. Some HiAPs are driven and owned by the health sector (Type 1), others are perhaps initiated, but co-owned with the health sector (Type 2), and some owned by other sectors with possible health sector input (Type 3).

In all cases there is a need for a clearer view of the drivers and barriers of sectoral thinking—this would enable the developer of these types of "interventions" to take action to blur boundaries and transcend siloed thinking. Concepts like joined-up-government, whole-of-government, government co-ordination, horizontal and integrated government and governance (echoing the intersectoral and HiAP rhetoric) have emerged from administrative and political science since the 1970s and have been attempted to be implemented in the public sector since the 1980s (through insights from

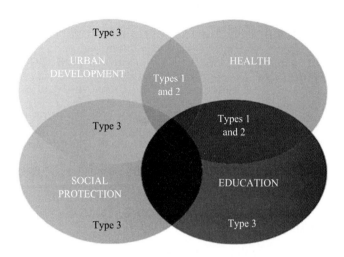

Fig.7 Types of interventions between and across sectoral realms[26]

governance and public administration science). Key notions to develop such comprehensive and coherent approaches (which Peters[27] calls the "Holy Grail" of public administration) relate to the idea of governance ("steering and co-ordinating a complex range of organizations via a control system constructed upon a multiplicity of linkages" [28]). The tools of good governance include control, coordination, accountability and power [25]. But most of all, governance for integration relates to politics [29]. It appears political systems (electorates, parliaments, the caste of Ministers and Secretaries, and political appointees) have failed to make integration a high priority—either because it is too complex and elusive, or because it would be a challenge to the very integrity of the political economy.

There is a degree of consensus, that barriers to integration at least include issues around existing fragmentation; (lack of) accountability; organisational departmentalism; and interpersonal relationships as well as leadership. Even where statutory requirements for integration exist—often legislative—approaches do not necessarily facilitate or enforce material—sometimes called substantive—policy development (beyond symbolic policy), that is, policy that dedicates resources accountably to resolving defined and attainable objectives.

In moving toward horizontal, integrated government Peters [27] identifies four pathways: through systems of participation for all stakeholders; through acknowledgement and institutionalisation of networking; through the establishment of coordination-targeted organisational behavioural values; and through extending the epistemic community to include all relevant stakeholder in knowledge creation and utilisation. Such rather abstract approaches may not necessarily lead to success, particularly as the area of integrated health policy is considered "a moving target" or a "complex adaptive system"[30]: "A collection of individual agents with freedom to act in ways that are not always totally predictable, and whose actions are interconnected so that one agent's actions changes the context for other agents."

The literature on integrated public sector efforts for health is little unequivocal in its conceptual development. Terms such as "intersectoral governance"[31], "intersectoral action"[32], "multisectoral action"[33], Healthy Public Policy and Health in All Policies are used interchangeably. In fact, whereas HiAP as a concept was codified in the outcome document of the WHO and Government of Finland 8th Global Conference on Health Promotion and its essential background documents[34], the relevant follow-up resolution of the World Health Assembly did not refer to HiAP front and centre, but rather described its scope as "a framework to promote action across sectors of health and health equity"[35]—this careful framing of the issue demonstrates how engagement toward integral approaches for health development is a politically challenging realm and deliberately obscured.

However, a conceptual distinction between (intersectoral, integrated, etc.) governance, policy and action is required, and we follow the relevant evidence on European Healthy Cities[36].

An overview is provided in Table 1. Intersectoral governance is "the sum of the many ways individuals and institutions, public and private, manage the connections of their common affairs. It is a continuing process through which conflicting or diverse interests may be accommodated and cooperative action may be taken. It includes formal institutions and regimes empowered to enforce compliance, as well as informal arrangements that people and institutions either have agreed to or perceive to be in their interest". Health governance is an often intangible set of values and beliefs on "how we do things around here" and a decisive definition is called for but not yet available. Three types of governance have been identified[37] that play out at multiple levels between social system and individual behaviour. Following De Leeuw, Clavier and Breton[38] intersectoral policy is "the expressed intent of government to allocate resources and capacities across relevant actors to resolve an expressly identified health issue within a certain timeframe". This happens in regulatory, distributive, or redistributive fashion. In conceptualising intersectoral action it seems useful to align "Action" with the policy instrument literature. Policy instruments "affect either the content or processes of policy implementation, that is, which alter the way goods and services are delivered to the public or the manner in which such implementation processes take place" [39] but they play a role across policy design from problem definition to outcome evaluation. Perhaps crudely, the intersectoral action toolbox consists of (positive and negative) sanctions, the creation of facilities, and communicative action.

Perhaps too crudely, "Governance" sets the overall rules for the game, "Policy" is the substantive decision to address a problem, and "Action" is the tool to make change happen.

Table 1 Typologies of (intersectoral) governance, policy and action (policy instruments) [24]

Governance	Policy	Action
Constitutive	Regulatory	Sanctions
Directive	Distributive	Facilities
Operational	Redistributive	Communication

Attempting to clarify these critical concepts should not obscure the fact that the empirical study of integrated governance, policy and action for health is a challenging enterprise. A first attempt to produce a systematic overview of health governance at the interface between levels of government across 46 member states of the European Region of WHO was produced in 1998 [40]. A follow-up descriptive inventory of 99 European cities was published in 2015 [41]. One thing becomes clear from this body of work: the sets of rules of the game, and how they relate between levels of government, is unique and specific for each particular setting—this presents challenges for systematic inquiry but novel methodologies are at hand, including Realist Synthesis[42].

4 Tools to develop HiAP

It is therefore not surprising that accounts of methods to engage for integrated health governance, policy and action are often cursory (based on a selection of particular case studies), abstract (based on theory and/or rhetoric) and missionary (instructions) in nature.

Two examples of training manuals and capacity building tools are relevant. WHO developed and validated a manual for HiAP development. The manual states:

"Given government responsibility for health and the complexity of many contemporary health challenges, governments have several crucial roles to play in the HiAP approach including but not limited to:

- commissioning research;
- engaging stakeholders within and beyond government;
- formulating and implementing intersectoral policies; and
- evaluating their impact."

The manual further adopts the recommendations by the "intersectoral governance" proponents that HiAP is supported by the establishment of (a combination of)

(1) cabinet committees and secretariats;

(2) parliamentary committees;

(3) interdepartmental committees and units;

(4) mega-ministries and merges;

(5) joint budgeting;

(6) intersectoral policy-making procedures;

(7) non-governmental stakeholder engagement.

To move toward the establishment and durability of such structures and approaches, the Manual adopts the typology of arguments for HiAP proposed by Leppo and colleagues [43]:

(1) the health argument—health is an intrinsic value and governments can and should support public sector engagement in health development.

(2) the health-to-other-sector argument—health and equity improvements can help achieve government mandates across the public sector.

(3) the health-societal-goal argument—health and equity development contribute to wider societal gain across social spheres.

(4) the economic argument—as identified earlier, health is good for wealth, and socio-economic growth.

Evidence also exists that indicates that the health argument may be counterproductive. Scottish respondents to a survey advise to avoid the H word— "health", and Healthy Cities seem to thrive intersectorally when the starting point is environmental sustainability rather than health.

We distinguished stages in the HiAP process, between initiation, coordination, and routinization, upon which different scholarly disciplinary and empirical perspectives were overlayed. The literature on HiAP places significant emphasis on leadership, not just of peak institutional bodies like Ministries, but also on the leadership of practitioners and communities [44]. As outlined above, there are a number of insightful analyses of concrete steps that can be taken to integrate governance, policy and action for health, notably generated through the World Health Organization, South Australia, and Finland. We outlined the multiple governance framework earlier in this piece and believe different kinds of institutions and "rules" can and should be applied to different levels of understanding to bring together often disparate perspectives. We have also found some case material that substantiates some of these views [45], and a critical level of understanding the possibilities of integrated policies for health lies in a better appreciation of the mechanisms at the nexus between research, policy and practice [46]. Ultimately, though, we see the development and sustainability of Health in All Policies as a matter of community action and engaged (political) leadership across the governance-policy-action spectrum, in which all different levels of institutional rule book need to be at least thought of, and possibly acted upon. "Top-down" needs to meet "bottom-up" and dynamic complexity needs to meet singularly focused analysis. The Holy Grail of Integration is within reach—we only need to put our minds to it.

References

[1]   MARMOT M. Social determinants of health inequalities. The Lancet, 2005, 365(9464):1099–1104.

[2]   BLUM H L. Planning for health: development and application of social change theory. Human Sciences Press. 1974.

[3]   LAFRAMBOISE H L. Health policy: breaking the problem down into more manageable segments. Canadian Medical Association Journal, 1973, 108(3):388.

[4]   EVANS R G, BARER M L, MARMOR T R. Why are some people healthy and others not? The determinants of the health of populations. Transaction Publishers. 1994.

[5]   ERIKSSON M, LINDSTRÖM B. Antonovsky's sense of coherence scale and the relation with health: a systematic review. Journal of Epidemiology & Community Health, 2006, 60(5):376–381.

[6]   DAHLGREN G, WHITEHEAD M. Policies and strategies to promote equity in health. World Health Organization, Regional Office for Europe. 1992.

[7]   GRAHAM H. Social determinants and their unequal distribution: clarifying policy understandings. The Milbank Quarterly, 2004, 82(1):101–124.

[8]   Canadian Council on Social Determinants of Health. A review of frameworks on the determinants of health. 2015.

[9]   MILIO N. Promoting health through public policy. Philadelphia: FA Davis Co. 1981.

［10］ HANCOCK T. Beyond health care: from public health policy to healthy public policy. Canadian Public Health Association, Ottawa.1985.

［11］ DE LEEUW E, CLAVIER C. Healthy public in all policies. Health Promotion International, 2011,26(suppl 2): ii237-244.

［12］ World Health Organization, Health Canada, Canadian Public Health Association. The Ottawa charter for health promotion: the move towards a new public health. 1986.

［13］ World Health Organization. Adelaide recommendations for healthy public policy. 1988.

［14］ NUTBEAM D. Health promotion glossary. Health Promotion International,1998,13:349-364.

［15］ FAFARD P. Evidence and healthy public policy: insights from health and political sciences. Canadian Policy Research Networks May. 2008.

［16］ MARMOR T R, BOYUM D. Medical care and public policy: the benefits and burdens of asking fundamental questions. Health Policy (Amsterdam, Netherlands),1999,49: 27-43.

［17］ HANCOCK T. Health promotion in Canada: 25 years of unfulfilled promise. Health Promotion International, 2011, 26(suppl 2): ii263-267.

［18］ DE LEEUW E, GREEN G, SPANSWICK L, et al. Policymaking in European healthy cities. Health Promotion International,2015,30: i18-31.

［19］ BOWMAN S, UNWIN N, CRITCHLEY J, et al. Use of evidence to support healthy public policy: a policy effectiveness-feasibility loop. Bulletin of the World Health Organization,2012,90:847-853.

［20］ BRETON E, DE LEEUW E. Theories of the policy process in health promotion research: a review. Health Promotion International,2011,26: 82-90.

［21］ World Health Organization. Intersectoral action for health: the role of intersectoral cooperation in national strategies for health for all.1986.

［22］ CHRISTENSEN T, LÆGREID P. The whole-of-government approach to public sector reform. Public Administration Review,2007,67: 1059-1066.

［23］ DE LEEUW E. Engagement of sectors other than health in integrated health governance, policy, and action. Annual Review of Public Health, 2017,38:329-349.

［24］ DE LEEUW E. From urban projects to healthy city policies//DE LEEUW E, SIMOS J. Healthy Cities—The Theory, Policy, and Practice of Value-based Urban Planning. Springer. 2017:407-437.

［25］ RUDOLPH L, CAPLAN J, BEN-MOSHE K, et al. Health in all policies: a guide for state and local governments. American Public Health Association and Public Health Institute. 2013.

［26］ WHO. The economics of the social determinants of health and health inequalities: a resource book. 2013.

［27］ PETERS B G. Managing horizontal government: the politics of co-ordination. Public Administration,1998,76: 295-311.

［28］ FLINDERS M. Governance in Whitehall. Public Administration,2002, 80: 51-75.

［29］ DE LEEUW E, PETERS D. Nine questions to guide development and implementation of Health in All Policies. Health Promotion International,2015,30: 987-997.

［30］ PLSEK P E, GREENHALGH T. Complexity science: the challenge of complexity in health care. BMJ,2001, 323: 625-628.

[31] MCQUEEN D, WISMAR M, LIN V, et al. Intersectoral governance for health in all policies: structures, actions and experiences. Copenhagen: World Health Organization Regional Office for Europe. 2012.

[32] MARMOT M, ALLEN J J. Social determinants of health equity. American Journal of Public Health, 2014, 104 (suppl 4): 517–519.

[33] World Health Organization. Global action plan for the prevention and control of noncommunicable diseases 2013–2020. 2013.

[34] PUSKA P, STÅHL T. Health in all policies—the finnish initiative: background, principles, and current issues. Annual review of public health, 2010, 31: 315–328.

[35] World Health Assembly. Resolution WHA67.12 Contributing to social and economic development: sustainable action across sectors to improve health and health equity. 2014.

[36] DE LEEUW E. Intersectoral action, policy and governance in European Healthy Cities. Public Health Panorama, 2015, 1(2): 175–182.

[37] HILL M, HUPE P. Analysing policy processes as multiple governance: accountability in social policy. Policy Politics, 2006, 34: 557–573.

[38] DE LEEUW E, CLAVIER C, BRETON E. Health policy—why research it and how: health political science. Health Research Policy and Systems, 2014, 12(1): 55.

[39] HOWLETT M. Managing the "hollow state": procedural policy instruments and modern governance. Canadian Public Administration. 2000: 412–431.

[40] GREEN G. Health and governance in European cities: a compendium of trends and responsibilities for public health in 46 member states of the WHO European Region. European Hospital Management Journal. 1988.

[41] DE LEEUW E, PALMER N, SPANSWICK L. City fact sheets: WHO European Healthy Cities Network. Copenhagen: World Health Organization Regional Office for Europe. 2015.

[42] DE LEEUW E, GREEN G, DYAKOVA M, et al. European healthy cities evaluation: conceptual framework and methodology. Health Promotion International, 2015, 30(suppl 1): i8–17.

[43] LEPPO K, OLLILA E, PENA S, et al. Health in all policies. Seizing Opportunities, Implementing Policies. Helsinki: Ministry of Social Affairs and Health. 2013.

[44] GREER S L, LILLYIS D F. Beyond leadership: political strategies for coordination in health policies. Health Policy, 2014, 116(1): 12–17.

[45] SHANKARDASS K, SOLAR O, MURPHY K, et al. A scoping review of intersectoral action for health equity involving governments. International Journal of Public Health, 2012, 57: 25–33.

[46] DE LEEUW E. From research to policy and practice in public health//LIAMPUTTONG P. Public Health: Local and Global Perspectives. Cambridge University Press, 2016: 213–234.

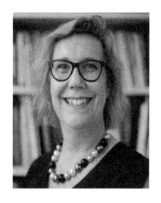

Eyelyne de Leeuw is the Director of CHETRE and Editor-in-Chief of *Health Promotion International*, former Director of the WHO Collaborating Centre for Research on Healthy Cities at the Maastricht University, Honorary Professor of Deakin University and La Trobe University, Visiting Professor of University of Montreal and Maastricht University, WHO European Research Director for Healthy Cities.

Better Health by 2030: *The Global Charter* and the Sustainable Development Goals

Michael Moore

World Federation of Public Health Associations

The Global Charter for the Public's Health [1] (*The Global Charter* for short) was developed by the World Federation of Public Health Associations (WFPHA) in collaboration with the World Health Organization (WHO) and a wide range of stakeholders. The intention of the Charter was to move away from specific disease focused policy and to provide guidance on improving health through " prevention, protection and health promotion ". In order to do this, the Charter identified four enablers: capacity building, good governance, information, and advocacy.

The Charter was designed to be considered in concert with the Sustainable Development Goal (SDGs) [2]. All nations, as members of the United Nations, have committed to implement the SDGs. As such, it is appropriate, therefore, to identify the importance of using the Charter as a pathway to assist in the implementation of these goals.

1　Protection

SDG 13: Protecting health from climate risks, and promoting health through low-carbon development

When Dr. Margaret Chan, as Director of the WHO, approached the WFPHA to develop the Charter, she expressed her concern about the broad challenges facing the goals of improving health. The huge challenges of improving health internationally needed not only appropriate action, but an appropriate framework for action. The Director General through down the gauntlet in her closing comments at the 130th session of the WHO Executive Board with the words "The challenges facing public health, and the broader world context in which we struggle, have become too numerous and too complex for a business-as-usual approach." [3]

Protection of health is one of the three center-pieces of the Charter.

1.1　International Health is a key element of the coordination between countries. Health has no borders. With this in mind international health regulations that are "an international legal instrument that is binding on 196 countries across the globe, including all the Member States of WHO" [4]. They provide an important aspect of the protection of populations that can only be achieved through appropriate coordination.

1.2　Communicable disease control is also an issue that knows no borders and the experience, influence and leadership of China in the "bird flu" and "swine flu" outbreaks has been a key element for international preparedness of countries in handling communicable diseases [5].

1.3　Emergency preparedness runs side by side with communicable disease preparedness. Lessons learnt from the Ebola outbreak in West Africa, tsunamis and earthquakes and other emergencies are stark reminders of what happens when there is a failure in having the capacity to handle emergencies.

1.4　Planetary health considerations are a key element of protection. The concept includes: environmental health, climate change, and sustainability. "Planetary health is the health of human civilization and the state of the natural systems on which it depends" [6].

1.5　One of the key elements of planetary health is climate action. Climate change provides one of the greatest challenges for the health of the international community.

1.5.1　Withdrawal from the Paris accord by President Trump citing "Pittsburgh not Paris" [7] seemed like a global disaster being perpetrated by one of the world's greatest polluters—the USA. However, it is important to keep in mind that there is strong movement at the local level within the USA with State governors and city mayors forming by June 2017 the US Climate Alliance with 10 States and 274 cities [8].

1.5.2　There is a similar story in the Pacific. Australia faced the threat of further coal mining with the Turnbull government proposing to support Indian businesses Adani in the development of a new coal mine at Carmichael that will be among the largest in the world [9]. The threats to climate action are a real and present danger.

1.5.3　In the meantime, small Pacific Nations will bear the brunt of the impact. At a meeting of the Intergovernmental Panel on Climate Change (IPCC) co-hosted by the

University of the South Pacific in Fiji there was concern with "the United Nations Framework Convention on Climate Change (UNFCCC) and the world at large, on how critical the problem is and how urgently the world needs to act to save our islands, our land, our people, cultures and ultimately our countries" [10].

2　Prevention

SDG 12: Responsible consumption and production

The Global Charter for the Public's Health considers that prevention ought to be seen broadly as incorporating: primary prevention—vaccination; secondary prevention—screening; tertiary prevention—evidence-based, community-based, integrated, person-centered quality health-care and rehabilitation; healthcare management and planning.

When examined in the light of the SDGs, the Charter's prevention focus may be considered in the light of SDG 12 "responsible consumption and production".

2.1　Anti-microbial resistance (AMR) has become an international challenge resulting, at least in part, from irresponsible consumption. In Australia predictions have been made that AMR will overtake cancer as the leading cause of mortality by 2050 [11]. The authors point out that "Given that bacteria do not respect international borders, AMR can spread rapidly and undetected and is, therefore, a global concern for all."

2.2　Other challenges for responsible consumption include tobacco, junk food and alcohol.

2.2.1　The Philip Morris tobacco company would have us believe it is a leopard that has changed its spots [12] arguing that it seeks a "tobacco free world". Whilst focusing on developing economies to push its lethal product (that when used as directed-kills two thirds of people ten years younger than those who do not smoke [13]) the company argues that the unproved e-Cigarettes and IQOS will deliver a tobacco-free world. The hypocrisy is frightening! Tobacco kills. Evidence of harm associated with drawing ultra-fine particles into the lungs through other devices remains at best equivocal.

2.2.2　Obesity remains an international challenge with a high risk that consumption pushed by international conglomerates will mean that the next generation, for the first time in recent centuries will live less healthy and shorter lives than the current generation.

2.2.3　The harmful use of alcohol is also a major challenge with unhealthy consumption feeding into the profits of international companies. Harmful use of alcohol results in a range of diseases from liver and cardiovascular disease to cancer. However, it is also a key catalyst in increasing violence both in public and at the domestic level.

2.3   Good government stewardship is required internationally if the health (or poor health) agenda is not to be set by international companies whose prime focus is profit rather than health. With regard to responsible consumption, good government stewardship means:

2.3.1   Promoting healthy consumption through appropriate marketing, accurate information and interventions such as effective labelling [14].

2.3.2   Restricting marketing of products known to be unhealthy is an important role for government. One example is the sponsorship of motor sport by alcohol companies. The harmful relationship between driving and alcohol is well known and this sort of marketing should simply be banned nationally and internationally.

2.3.3   Resisting arguments about the "nanny state" [15] are also important for public health. It is far better to have interventions and tone set by government rather than allowing major international companies to set the health agenda.

3   Health promotion

SDG 1: Prioritizing the health needs of the poor
SDG 10: Reduce inequalities

Health Promotion is set out in the Charter in a broad context that draws from the *Ottawa Charter* and builds on more recent updates. It includes issues such as: inequalities; environmental determinants; social and economic determinants; resilience; behavior and health literacy; life-course; and healthy settings.

3.1   Within the WHO "Health in the SDG Era" SDG 1 refers to "prioritizing the health needs of the poor" and SDG 10 to "reduce inequalities". These a key elements in terms of implementation of the Charter. The evidence that the world is moving in the opposite direction, unfortunately, is overwhelming with the rich getting richer and the poor getting poorer. Growing disparity internationally, nationally and locally must be a key challenge for those interested in improving health outcomes for all. An Oxfam reported of January 2017 and other reports on wealth inequality provide a stark warning [16].

3.1.1   Internationally, even one outstanding revelation provides a clear picture of the challenges. "Just eight billionaires have wealth equal to the poorest three point six billion people". In Australia, there is a similar story where "one percent of Australians own equivalent wealth to the bottom seventy percent".

3.1.2   Globally, "one in ten people survive on less than two dollars per day".

3.2   Oxfam international were clear in showing "how, in order to maximize returns to their wealthy shareholders, big corporations are dodging taxes, driving down wages for their workers and the prices paid to producers, and investing less in their business".

4   Good governance

SDG 3: Good health and well-being

The Charter sets out the key elements of good governance for equitable health outcomes. They include: public health legislation; health and cross-sector policy; strategy; financing; organization; assurance; transparency; and accountability and audit. When examining "Health in the SDG Era" the central thrust is a focus on SDG 3 "good health and well-being".

These may be divided into challenges and hopes.

4.1   Challenges

4.1.1   Challenges include maternal mortality. Whilst internationally maternal mortality has improved considerably over the last fifty years, this has not been shared equitably and there remain considerable numbers of communities that have very poor health outcomes for birthing mothers.

4.1.2   HIV/AIDS, tuberculosis (including anti-biotic resistant forms), malaria and many other diseases still provide desperate challenges internationally. However, the major challenge for these diseases remains the underlying issue of poverty. Fundamental to public health is an understanding of the social determinants of health.

4.1.3   Non-communicable diseases are on the rise. Obesity is no longer associated with developed economies. Low and middle income countries are now experiencing considerable increases with the associated costs in health care, increased morbidity and mortality. This challenge is identified as a "Tsunami of obesity" that "threatens all regions of the world" [17].

4.1.4   Morbidity and mortality associated with road accidents are reducing in developed countries but are on the increase in low and middle income countries. Methods of dealing with this health burden are known and need to be implemented.

4.2 Hopes

4.2.1　The Framework Convention on Tobacco Control provides a clear direction for dealing with disease and death associated with smoking tobacco. Australians are amongst the lowest users of tobacco in the world. In 2016, just 2% of teenagers were non-smokers while amongst Australians of all ages there were only 12% who were daily smokers [19]. Multi-faceted approaches to reducing smoking that have been adopted in some countries may be extrapolated to others where high prevalence of smoking remains.

4.2.2　Vaccination continues to be one of the most effective methods of tackling infectious disease. Smallpox has been eliminated through immunization and the world stands on the brink of eliminating polio. The coordinated global effort of Rotary International, the WHO, GAVI, Gates Foundation along with governments other NGOs and individuals means that progress is being made. In December the number of cases of infection with wild polio virus in 2017 more than halved from the previous year down to just seventeen cases [19].

4.2.3　International treaties have a major impact on health. Although many challenges remain, the issues were identified by the World Trade Organization in 2001. The *Doha Declaration* attempted to deal with "the need for governments to apply the principles of public health and the terms of the Agreement on Trade-related Aspects of Intellectual Property Rights (TRIPS [20])". One of the key elements was to identify ways to ensure more equitable access to essential medicines and health products.

5 Accurate information

SDG 4：Supporting high-quality education for all to improve health and equity

The Charter provides an insight into the importance and influence of accurate information. In public health terms this means ensuring engagement with surveillance, monitoring and evaluation; monitoring of health determinants; research and evidence; risk and innovation; dissemination and uptake.

5.1　The example taken from the Health in the SDG Era diagram is SDG four which seeks to support "high-quality education for all to improve health and equity". In the context of the Charter, it is critical that decision making is based on the best possible evidence.

5.2   Not only is evidence critical but the importance of explaining health policy so that it is communicated across all sectors of the community is also vital. Open public health debates, when based on evidence, help to dispel myths on issues such as vaccination and unhealthy activities such as gambling along with unhealthy consumption of tobacco, alcohol and junk food.

5.3   Such debates provide the opportunity to identify the economic costs of failure of public health policy and the impact not only on the health of people but on the productivity and gross domestic product of nations.

5.4   Monitoring and evaluation also forms a key role in measuring success. In the words of former WHO Director General Dr. Margaret Chan, "As I often say, what gets measured gets done".

5.5   Monitoring, however, is not enough. The use of traditional and social media to spread healthy messages has become a critical element in public health. Companies that promote unhealthy activities and commodities are now using such methods extensively and need to be countered for a healthy future by 2030.

6   Capacity building

SDG 6: Clean water and sanitation

Capacity building in public health is a key element of improving health internationally. The concept puts responsibility on governments, NGOs, universities and other education institutions and all public health professionals. The Charter identifies key areas of capacity building as: workforce development for public health, health workers and wider workforce; workforce planning; numbers, resources, infrastructure; standards, curriculum, accreditation; capabilities, teaching and training.

6.1   The example used with regard to capacity building is Health in the SDG Era goal six "Clean water and sanitation". This goal is basic. Students of public health and epidemiology are exposed to this issue as one of the first parts of their course of study.

6.2   The story of John Snow and the reverend Henry Whitehead conducting the first British epidemiological study forms the first chapter of many epidemiology texts [21]. However, the texts tend to stop at the discovery of cholera spread through the Broad Street pump. The part of the often untold story is that, whilst their evidence was used by the British government to introduce sewers to London and throughout the country, the catalyst for action was actually the "Great Stink" of London in 1858. The Parliament of

Westminster was unable to meet as the smell was simply overwhelming. Under the circumstances the Members of Parliament used the evidence and found a way to take action. The message is clear—public health is political.

6.3　A joint report by WHO/UNICEF [22] in 2017 suggests that "in 90 countries, progress towards basic sanitation is too slow, meaning they will not reach universal coverage by 2030". Furthermore, "Some 3 in 10 people worldwide, or 2.1 billion, lack access to safe, readily available water at home, and 6 in 10, or 4.5 billion, lack safely managed sanitation"

6.4　We have known for more than one and a half centuries how important clean water and sanitation are for health—and yet capacity has not been there to deliver. Political action is needed to move forward.

7　Effective advocacy

SDG 17: Mobilizing partners to monitor and attain health related SDGs

Effective Advocacy has been identified by the WFPHA as a key enabler for better health. Effective advocacy goes well beyond "lobbying". It encompasses: leadership and ethics; health equity; social-mobilization and solidarity; education of the public; people-centered approach; voluntary community sector engagement; communications; and, sustainable development.

7.1　Mobilizing partners to monitor and attain health and related SDGs is the final example that will be cited from the "Health in the SDG Era".

7.2　The World Federation of Public Health Associations (WFPHA) has over 120 member associations worldwide and works with a wide range of stakeholders to bring about better health outcomes internationally. This represents over a million people globally with a keen interest in public health. The vision of the WFPHA is to "lead the quest for health equity and a long and healthy life for all people". The mission is an "international, non-governmental, civil society, multi-disciplinary federation of public health associations dedicated to preventing disease, and the promotion and protection of the public's health".

7.3　The Chinese Preventive Medicine Association (CPMA) is a member of the WFPHA and was established thirty years ago and has been involved in considerable influence for better health outcomes not just in China but across the Western Pacific and internationally. The CPMA has taken on responsibility for the Western Pacific Region of the WFPHA and has engaged with public health associations throughout the region facilitating networking, capacity building and advocacy where appropriate.

7.4 The CPMA has also been an active member of the Governing Council of the WFPHA encouraging better health outcomes through effective policies and sensible engagement.

7.5 The WFPHA is in formal relations with the WHO. The development of the Charter grew out of this relationship and many other opportunities are presented to the WFPHA and its members associations through this and many other relationships. One of the key elements of effective advocacy is managing relationships for influence[23].

8 Conclusions

China has achieved extraordinary improvements in health over the 30 years since the formation of the Chinese Preventive Medicine Association. However, so much more can be done to ensure equity in health outcomes, to improve prevention and protection and to strengthen health promotion. To achieve better protection, prevention and health promotion as a method of implementing the SDGs, public health associations, governments and industry can use a range of important tools. These tools have been identified in the Charter as: good governance, capacity building, accurate information, and advocacy.

The examples used above illustrate the relationship between the Charter and the SDGs. However, they are a selection of examples. The Charter has the potential to be used as a method of implementation across a much broader range of the SDGs. Considering the commitment of governments globally to implement the SDGs, the Charter provides one tool that could be used to assist in their implementation.

References

[1] LOMAZZI M A. Global charter for the public's health—the public health system: role, functions, competencies and education requirements. Eur J Public Health,2016,26(2): 210-212.

[2] UN. Sustainable Development Goals 2017. 2017.

[3] CHAN M. WHO Director General Addresses the Executive Board. 2012.

[4] WHO. International Health Regulations 2007. 2017.

[5] YANG W Z. Early warning for infectious disease outbreak theory and practice. London: Elsevier ,2017.

[6] HORTON R, LO S. Planetary health: a new science for exceptional action. Lancet,2015,386(10007):1921-1922.

[7] WATTS M. Cities spearhead climate action. Nature Climate Change,2017,7:537-538.

[8] MINDOCK C. Paris agreement: US states and mayors fight climate change after Donald Trump pulls US out of deal. 2017.

[9] HOLMES D. Australia's climate bomb: the senselessness of Adani's Carmichael coal mine. 2017.

[10] University of the South Pacific. USP co-hosts Fiji's inaugural Lead Authors Meeting for IPCC. 2017.

[11] KELLY R, DAVIES S C. Tackling antimicrobial resistance globally. Med J Aust, 2017,207(9):371-373.

[12] WHO. WHO statement on Philip Morris funded foundation for a smoke-free world. 2017.

[13] BANKS E, JOSHYG, WEBER M F, et al. Tobacco smoking and all-cause mortality in a large Australian cohort study: findings from a mature epidemic with current low smoking prevalence. BMC Medicine,2015,13(1):38.

[14] TALATI Z,NORMAN R,PETTIGREW S, et al. The impact of interpretive and reductive front-of-pack labels on food choice and willingness to pay. International Journal of Behavioral Nutrition and Physical Activity,2017,14(1):171.

[15] MOORE M, YEATMAN H DAVEY R. Which nanny—the state or industry? Wowsers, teetotallers and the fun police in public health advocacy. Public Health, 2015,129(8):1030-1037.

[16] Oxfam International. An economy for the 99 percent. 2017.

[17] WISE J. "Tsunami of obesity" threatens all regions of world, researchers find. BMJ,2011, 342:772.

[18] AIHW. Teenage smoking and drinking down, while drug use rises among older people. 2017.

[19] GPEI. Polio global eradication initiative. 2017.

[20] WHO. The Doha declaration on the TRIPS agreement and public health. 2017.

[21] HENNEKENS C H, BURING J E. Epidemiology in medicine. Little Brown and Company,1987.

[22] WHO/UNICEF. Progress on drinking water, sanitation and hygiene: 2017 update and sustainable development goal. 2017.

[23] MOORE M, YEATMAN H, POLLARD C. Evaluating success in public health advocacy strategies. Vietnam Journal of Public Health,2013,1(1):66-75.

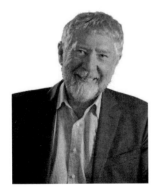

Michael Moore is the CEO of the Public Health Association of Australia, the President of the World Federation of Public Health Associations, Former Minister of Health and Community Care, Independent Member of the Australian Capital Territory Legislative Assembly (1989-2001), Member of the Order of Australia (AM), Visiting Professor at the University of Technology Sydney, Adjunct Professor with the University of Canberra.

后　　记

科学技术是第一生产力。纵观历史,人类文明的每一次进步都是由重大的科学发现与技术革命所引领和支撑的。进入 21 世纪,科学技术日益成为经济社会发展的主要驱动力。我们国家的发展必须以科学发展为主题,以加快转变经济发展方式为主线。而实现科学发展、加快转变经济发展方式,最根本的是要依靠科技的力量,最关键的是要大幅提高自主创新能力,要推动我国经济社会发展尽快走上创新驱动的轨道。党的十八大报告指出,科技创新是提高社会生产力和综合国力的重要支撑,必须摆在国家发展全局的核心位置,要实施"创新驱动发展战略"。

面对未来发展的重任,中国工程院将进一步发挥院士作用,邀请世界顶级专家参与,共同以国际视野和战略思维开展学术交流与研讨,为国家战略决策提供科学思想和系统方案,以科学咨询支持科学决策,以科学决策引领科学发展。

只有高瞻远瞩,才能统筹协调、突出重点地建设好国家创新体系。工程院历来高度重视中长期工程科技发展战略研究,通过对未来 20 年及至更长远的工程科技发展前景进行展望与规划,做好顶层设计,推动我国经济社会发展尽快走上创新驱动的轨道。

自 2011 年起,中国工程院开始举办一系列国际工程科技发展战略高端论坛,旨在为相关领域的中外顶级专家搭建高水平高层次的国际交流平台,通过开展宏观性、战略性、前瞻性的研究,进一步认识和把握工程科技发展的客观规律,从而更好地引领未来工程科技的发展。

中国工程院学术与出版委员会将国际工程科技发展战略高端论坛的报告汇编出版。仅以此编之作聚百家之智,汇学术前沿之观点,为人类工程科技发展贡献一份力量。

中国工程院